Long Cases in G
Medicine

Edited by R.E. Pounder MA, MD, FRCP

Reader in Medicine and
Honorary Consultant Gastroenterologist,
The Royal Free Hospital School of Medicine and
The Royal Free Hospital, London

SECOND EDITION

BLACKWELL SCIENTIFIC PUBLICATIONS

OXFORD LONDON EDINBURGH
BOSTON MELBOURNE

© 1983, 1989 by
Blackwell Scientific Publications
Editorial offices:
Osney Mead, Oxford OX2 0EL
    (Orders: Tel. 0865 240201)
8 John Street, London WC1N 2ES
23 Ainslie Place, Edinburgh EH3 6AJ
3 Cambridge Center, Suite 208
    Cambridge, Massachusetts
    02142, USA
107 Barry Street, Carlton
    Victoria 3053, Australia

First published 1983
Reprinted 1986, 1987
Second edition 1989

Set by Colset Private Ltd, Singapore
Printed and bound in Great Britain
by Billings of Worcester

DISTRIBUTORS

USA
    Year Book Medical Publishers
    200 North LaSalle Street,
    Chicago, Illinois 60601
    (Orders: Tel. 312–726–9733)

Canada
    The C.V. Mosby Company
    5240 Finch Avenue East
    Scarborough, Ontario
    (Orders: Tel. 416–298–1588)

Australia
    Blackwell Scientific Publications
    (Australia) Pty Ltd
    107 Barry Street
    Carlton, Victoria 3053
    (Orders: Tel. 03–347–0300)

British Library
Cataloguing in Publication Data

Long cases in general
    medicine—2nd ed
    1. Medicine—Questions &
    answers—For general practice
    I. Pounder, R.E. (Roy E.)
    610'.76

ISBN 0-632-02357-0

Contents

List of contributors

P. DANDONA DPhil MRCP, Senior Lecturer in Chemical Pathology and Director of the Metabolic Unit, The Royal Free Hospital School of Medicine, and The Royal Free Hospital, London.

D.G. GIBSON FRCP, Consultant Cardiologist, The Brompton Hospital, London.

G.R.V. HUGHES MD, FRCP, Consultant Physician, Department of Rheumatology, St Thomas's Hospital, and Head, Lupus Arthritis Research Unit, The Rayne Institute, St Thomas's Hospital, London.

D.G. JAMES MA, MD, FRCP, Adjunct Professor of Medicine, The Royal Free Hospital School of Medicine, London.

G.G. LLOYD MA, MD, MPhil, FRCPE, FRCPsych, Consultant Psychiatrist, The Royal Free Hospital, London.

E.J. PARKER-WILLIAMS FRCPath, Postgraduate Sub-Dean, Senior Lecturer in Haematology and Honorary Consultant Haematologist, St George's Hospital Medical School and St George's Hospital, London.

R.E. POUNDER MA, MD, FRCP, Reader in Medicine and Honorary Consultant Gastroenterologist, The Royal Free Hospital School of Medicine, and The Royal Free Hospital, London.

R.W. ROSS RUSSELL MA, MD, FRCP, Consultant Physician and Neurologist, The National Hospital for Nervous Diseases and St Thomas' Hospital, London.

DAME SHEILA SHERLOCK DBE, MD, FRCP, Consulting Physician, The Royal Free Hospital School of Medicine, and The Royal Free Hospital, London.

P. SWENY MA, MD, FRCP, Senior Lecturer in Medicine and Honorary Consultant Nephrologist, The Royal Free Hospital School of Medicine, and The Royal Free Hospital, London.

M.J. WALPORT MA, PhD MRCP, Senior Lecturer in Medicine and Honorary Consultant Rheumatologist, The Royal Postgraduate Medical School and Hammersmith Hospital, London

Preface to the second edition

This is the second and revised edition of *Long Cases in General Medicine*, which was first published six years ago. The book has been received enthusiastically by both undergraduate and postgraduate students, particularly because of its innovative style, and the fact that it shows how to present and discuss a clinical problem using a high standard of English.

Each of the original cases has been reviewed and brought up to date for this edition. It is interesting to see how clinical medicine has changed over the last six years — the major advances have been in infectious diseases and the more frequent use of sophisticated technology. I am also pleased to introduce a new contributor — Dr Geoffrey Lloyd who has prepared four interesting psychiatric cases for this edition.

The layout of the book is unchanged from the first edition. The histories are described in *Part 1: The Patient*, which provides clinical pictures and screening test results of 57 patients with general medical problems. In *Part 2: The Viva*, the reader is asked a series of questions:

What is the differential diagnosis?

What further investigations would you consider?

What is the final diagnosis?

How would you manage this patient?

The 11 contributors provide model answers to these questions, but the order of the cases has been rearranged to discourage cheating! Each contributor makes a final comment about the clinical problem, and then asks five follow-up questions, some of which are rather obscure, but can be answered by the use of an appropriate text book.

Finally , I would again like to thank Blackwell Scientific Publications, in particular Mr Peter Saugman and Ms Karen McNaught for their help in preparing this edition of *Long Cases in General Medicine*. I would like to thank my secretary Mrs Julia Young, succeeded by Ms Doris Elliott, who administered the revision of this edition. Finally, I would like to thank my wife Dr Christine Lee, and Jeremy and Tom, who on this occasion allowed me to take the paperwork away on holiday.

Roy Pounder
London, 1988

Preface to the first edition

Long Cases in General Medicine has a format that is unashamedly based upon the clinical stages of either the Final MB examination or the Membership examination of the Royal College of Physicians.

Why use this format? Firstly, the succession of questions that are posed about each patient in this book provides a logical system for diagnosis, investigation and management that can be carried into everyday clinical practice. Secondly, Long Cases provides the opportunity to discuss management decisions about common clinical problems, in a way that is not found in ordinary medical textbooks. Thirdly, examinations have a special way of concentrating the mind.

The histories described in Part 1: The Patient provide the clinical picture and screening test results of 53 patients with general medical problems. Their illnesses may be in any of nine specialities: Endocrinology, Cardiology, Respiratory Medicine, Hepatology, Gastroenterology, Rheumatology, Nephrology, Neurology or Haematology.

In Part 2: The Viva, the reader is asked a series of questions:
What is the differential diagnosis?
What further investigations would you consider?
What is the final diagnosis?
How would you manage this patient?

Ten contributors provide model answers to these questions, but the order of the cases has been re-arranged to discourage cheating. All the contributors work in teaching hospitals and have considerable experience on both sides of the examination desk. Each makes a final comment about the clinical problem and then asks five follow-up questions — the reader can search standard textbooks for the answers!

I hope that Long Cases in General Medicine will provide stimulating and informative reading for the clinical student as he or she approaches the Final MB examination. Long Cases should also be particularly helpful for candidates taking most higher medical examinations. Although the book is particularly relevant for the Membership examination of the Royal College of Physicians, it should also be helpful for pathologists, radiologists, anaesthetists and even, perhaps, surgeons in training.

The clinical problems in Long Cases are discussed very fully, providing up-to-date facts about the many illnesses raised in each differential diagnosis. I hope that the book will provide a stimulating new method for learning about General Medicine, whilst sitting in the armchair.

My thanks mainly go to the contributors whose opinions have fitted into the rather unusual format so successfully. I also thank Mr Adam

Sisman, of Blackwell Scientific Publications, whose enthusiasm remained throughout the months of preparation, and my secretary, Miss Julia Semus, who has cheerfully worked on the project from its very beginning. Finally I thank my wife, Christine, who tolerated all the paperwork at home and took Jeremy and Tom on holiday at a critical moment — but for that there would be no book!

Roy Pounder
London, 1983

How to use this book

1   Choose a case from *Part 1: The Patient*.

2   When you have read the history and seen the screening test results, which should be compared with the normal ranges shown below, answer these questions:
> What is the differential diagnosis?
> What further investigations would you consider?
> What is the final diagnosis?
> How would you manage this patient?

3   Turn to *Part 2: The Viva* and read the model answers written by experts.

4   Think about the follow-up questions, using a textbook to check your answers.

Screening tests — normal ranges

Haemoglobin		ESR	
male	13.0–18.0 g/dl	male	$< (\dfrac{\text{age in yrs}}{2})$ mm/1st hr
female	11.5–16.5 g/dl	female	$< (\dfrac{\text{age in yrs} + 10}{2})$ mm/1st hr
WBC	4.0–11.0×10^9/l	MCV	77–93 fl
Potassium	3.5–5.0 mmol/l	Sodium	135–145 mmol/l
Bicarbonate	24–32 mmol/l	Chloride	95–105 mmol/l
Urea	3.0–6.5 mmol/l	Creatinine	35–120 μmol/l
Calcium	2.10–2.60 mmol/l	Phosphate	0.70–1.25 mmol/l
Total Protein	60–80 g/l	Albumin	30–50 g/l
Bilirubin	5–17 μmol/l		
Aspartate Transaminase	5–40 U/l	Alkaline Phosphatase	35–130 U/l

Part 1: The Patient

Jaundice in a sauna secretary

An unmarried 29-year-old secretary worked for a sauna-owner. She presented with a rash on the face, malaise, nausea, weakness, anorexia, jaundice, dark urine and pale stools. She had never been jaundiced before, and had no contact with jaundiced persons. She had taken an oral contraceptive for nine years, but it was stopped with the onset of these symptoms. She did not abuse drugs. Five years ago she had silicone breast implants.

She started taking social amounts of alcohol at the age of 16. For the past five years she had been taking one and a half bottles of Martini (vermouth) daily and occasional spirits (about 160 g of alcohol daily). For eight months she had taken a drink before breakfast, and noticed nausea and tremor if she abstained.

On examination she was very ill and markedly jaundiced. She had a fever of 38.5°C. She weighed 52 kg and there was marked wasting of proximal limb muscles. There were florid spider naevi on the skin, most marked on the face, necklace area and arms. The palms were blotchy and red. The outstretched hands showed a flapping tremor, but a fine tremor was also present. The blood pressure was 150/80, pulse 120/min, with a systolic flow murmur over the apex of the heart. In the abdomen, a tender, smooth liver could be palpated 8 cm below the costal margin. A bruit could not be heard over it. The spleen was not palpable. There was mild ascites but no peripheral oedema. Focal neurological signs could not be elicited.

Screening test results

Haemoglobin	14.0 g/dl	ESR	50 mm/1st hr
WBC	25.7×10^9/l	MCV	106 fl
Potassium	3.2 mmol/l	Sodium	132 mmol/l
Bicarbonate	23 mmol/l	Chloride	94 mmol/l
Urea	5.0 mmol/l	Creatinine	92 μmol/l
Calcium	2.37 mmol/l	Phosphate	1.12 mmol/l
Total Protein	60 g/l	Albumin	34 g/l
Bilirubin	412 μmol/l		
Aspartate		Alkaline	
Transaminase	185 U/l	Phosphatase	15 U/l

Urine analysis: urobilinogen + + + +; bilirubin −

The Viva: questions and answers on page 117.

Depression and pleurisy

A nursing sister aged 27 complained of increasing malaise, intermittent pyrexias and bilateral pleuritic chest pains which had developed over the previous nine months. She had become depressed and irritable. She had missed much work, especially around the time of her menstrual periods when her symptoms became worse. After a 12-year pain-free interval migrainous headaches, which had troubled her as a child, had returned.

At the age of 12 she had developed a purpuric rash, and idiopathic thrombocytopenic purpura had been diagnosed. This had responded to corticosteroid therapy, but after a relapse splenectomy was performed when she was aged 14. Following this, purpura did not recur and she required no drug therapy.

On examination her temperature was 38.5°C. The skin over both elbows was erythematous and livedo reticularis was present on her limbs. The respiratory and cardiovascular systems were normal; there were no pleural or pericardial friction rubs, nor were any cardiac murmurs heard. Apart from a splenectomy scar her abdomen was normal. Both optic fundi were normal, and no abnormalities were found in her nervous system.

Screening test results

Haemoglobin	11.4 g/dl	ESR	97 mm/1st hr
WBC	3.9×10^9/l	MCV	86 fl
Potassium	4.6 mmol/l	Sodium	138 mmol/l
Bicarbonate	25 mmol/l	Chloride	103 mmol/l
Urea	4.2 mmol/l	Creatinine	88 μmol/l
Calcium	2.42 mmol/l	Phosphate	0.94 mmol/l
Total Protein	84 g/l	Albumin	40 g/l
Bilirubin	12 μmol/l		
Aspartate		Alkaline	
Transaminase	20 U/l	Phosphatase	60 U/l

Urine analysis: normal

The Viva: questions and answers on page 213.

Diarrhoea and abdominal pain

A 34-year-old research pharmacologist presented with a short history of diarrhoea and abdominal pain. For some years he had noticed occasional looseness of the bowels, but he became acutely ill six weeks before presentation. He was opening his bowels up to six times a day; at times the stools contained mucus and occasionally blood. The colicky abdominal pain was in the mid-abdomen, and was associated with mild distention and audible borborygmi. The patient became anorexic and his weight dropped from 65 to 61 kg. As he had a mild fever, his family doctor prescribed a five-day course of amoxycillin, without benefit. There had been no recent travel abroad, but three years earlier the patient had travelled extensively in Africa.

On examination the patient appeared pale and unwell. He had a temperature of 37.4°C. The abdomen was diffusely tender, slightly distended, with some fullness in the right iliac fossa. There were fleshy perianal skin tags; rectal examination was painful because of an anal fissure. Sigmoidoscopy revealed an erythematous rectal mucosa, without ulceration or haemorrhage.

Screening test results

Haemoglobin	11.0 g/dl	ESR	66 mm/1st hr
WBC	10.3×10^9/l	MCV	80 fl
Potassium	3.6 mmol/l	Sodium	140 mmol/l
Bicarbonate	28 mmol/l	Chloride	101 mmol/l
Urea	4.4 mmol/l	Creatinine	87 μmol/l
Calcium	2.28 mmol/l	Phosphate	0.72 mmol/l
Total Protein	66 g/l	Albumin	29 g/l
Bilirubin	5 μmol/l		
Aspartate		Alkaline	
Transaminase	18 U/l	Phosphatase	76 U/l

Urine analysis: normal

The Viva: questions and answers on page 95.

Oedema

A 33-year-old unmarried man was admitted to hospital with a three-month history of increasing oedema. In childhood he suffered a severe and deforming arthritis, requiring numerous hospital admissions. For five days he had noticed a reduction in his urinary output. He had been taking prednisolone 7.5 mg daily for the last 10 years.

On examination he looked unwell and was grossly oedematous with pitting oedema in the ankles, legs and thighs. There was marked sacral oedema. His upper limbs were thin and he appeared wasted despite the oedema. The JVP was not raised. His blood pressure was 120/60 lying and 90/55 standing. His feet were cold. The pulse was 80 and regular. There was dullness at both lung bases. Examination of his joints revealed a widespread and advanced deforming arthritis, with subluxation of the joints of both hands. Feet, ankles, elbows and knees were also affected, but to a lesser extent. Although tender and painful on movement, the joints were not hot or inflamed. The abdomen was distended with ascites. The spleen was just palpable and the liver was enlarged 2 cm below the costal margin.

Screening test results

Haemoglobin	7.9 g/dl	ESR	98 mm/1st hr
WBC	8.4 × 10^9/l	MCV	81 fl
Potassium	4.3 mmol/l	Sodium	133 mmol/l
Bicarbonate	22 mmol/l	Chloride	95 mmol/l
Urea	14.0 mmol/l	Creatinine	80 μmol/l
Calcium	1.91 mmol/l	Phosphate	1.10 mmol/l
Total Protein	56 g/l	Albumin	17 g/l
Bilirubin	4 μmol/l		
Aspartate		Alkaline	
Transaminase	19 U/l	Phosphatase	69 U/l

Urine analysis: protein + + + + ; blood +

The Viva: questions and answers on page 138.

Chinatown blues

A 53-year-old man from Hong Kong was working in a restaurant as a chef. He had left his family behind in Hong Kong, and was living in a lodging house. He felt lonely and depressed. He had attended a herbalist who had failed to eradicate his cough or to restore his potency. The patient was losing weight and felt generally unwell. He continued to smoke 40 cigarettes each day, but drank alcohol only moderately.

On examination the patient expectorated purulent sputum. He was emaciated and had finger clubbing. There was bronchial breathing in the right upper zone. The remainder of the physical examination was normal; in particular, there was no evidence of diabetes-associated cardiovascular, retinal or neurological disease.

Screening test results

Haemoglobin	9.7 g/dl	ESR	76 mm/1st hr
WBC	4.7×10^9/l	MCV	87 fl
Potassium	4.2 mmol/l	Sodium	139 mmol/l
Bicarbonate	29 mmol/l	Chloride	100 mmol/l
Urea	6.4 mmol/l	Creatinine	67 μmol/l
Calcium	2.59 mmol/l	Phosphate	0.81 mmol/l
Total Protein	77 g/l	Albumin	37 g/l
Bilirubin	15 μmol/l		
Aspartate Transaminase	21 U/l	Alkaline Phosphatase	60 U/l

Urine analysis: glucose + +

The Viva: questions and answers on page 223.

Eye problems

A 35-year-old secretary presented with a rapidly progressive prominence of her eyes. Over the previous six months she had suffered from marked irritation of the eyes, and had noticed some blurring of vision. For two years she had slowed up, noticing increased sensitivity to cold weather and some increase of weight.

15 years before she had been seen at another hospital for anxiety, weight loss, marked heat intolerance and profuse sweating. A surgeon had operated on her neck and her symptoms had subsided promptly. The patient's mother had pernicious anaemia and a maternal aunt was diabetic.

Examination revealed an obese, hypertensive patient with marked exophthalmos, exposure keratitis, periorbital oedema and inability to close her eyes completely. She had a pulse rate of 60/min in sinus rhythm. Her skin was dry, and localised areas of skin in front of the shin were thickened and hairy.

Screening test results

Haemoglobin	12.1 g/dl	ESR	10 mm/1st hr
WBC	$6.5 \times 10^9/l$	MCV	102 fl
Potassium	3.6 mmol/l	Sodium	132 mmol/l
Bicarbonate	24 mmol/l	Chloride	95 mmol/l
Urea	3.4 mmol/l	Creatinine	53 μmol/l
Calcium	2.35 mmol/l	Phosphate	1.12 mmol/l
Total Protein	77 g/l	Albumin	37 g/l
Bilirubin	10 μmol/l		
Aspartate		Alkaline	
Transaminase	28 U/l	Phosphatase	80 U/l

Urine analysis: glucose +

The Viva: questions and answers on page 178.

8

A painful eye

A 54-year-old woman developed sudden severe pain behind the right eye whilst doing housework. She went to bed and vomited 15 minutes later. The pain was partially relieved by aspirin but she remained in bed for one day. There was no fever. The following day she noticed diplopia and was found to have a ptosis on the right side. There was a past history of hypertension treated with bendrofluazide.

On examination there was limitation of adduction, elevation and depression of the right eye. The pupil was dilated and failed to react to light, either direct or consensual. Blood pressure was 180/105. An appointment was arranged with an ophthalmologist.

She rested at home for eight days, but then developed a sudden severe pain in the neck whilst straining at stool. She again vomited and over the next half-hour became drowsy. She was admitted to hospital later that day. Her blood pressure was 220/120, there was neck stiffness, and haemorrhages in both retinae. No lateralising signs were found in the nervous system, but the tendon reflexes were depressed and both plantar responses were extensor.

Screening test results

Haemoglobin	14.0 g/dl	ESR	16 mm/1st hr
WBC	12.0×10^9/l	MCV	89 fl
Potassium	3.8 mmol/l	Sodium	138 mmol/l
Bicarbonate	25 mmol/l	Chloride	101 mmol/l
Urea	6.2 mmol/l	Creatinine	98 μmol/l
Calcium	2.40 mmol/l	Phosphate	0.81 mmol/l
Total Protein	64 g/l	Albumin	36 g/l
Bilirubin	6 μmol/l		
Aspartate		Alkaline	
Transaminase	20 U/l	Phosphatase	40 U/l

Urine analysis: glucose + +

The Viva: questions and answers on page 190.

The dangers of exercise

A 32-year-old accountant was admitted after having collapsed whilst jogging. Over the previous year he had noted vague retrosternal pain, unrelated to exertion. On the day of admission he had developed more severe retrosternal pain while exercising, and had attempted to run through it. However, the pain became more severe and he fell to the ground, losing consciousness for a few minutes. There were no epileptic features.

As a child, a systolic murmur had been heard during an upper respiratory infection, and the possibility of rheumatic fever had been raised. His father had died suddenly at the age of 40 with a heart attack.

On examination he looked well. He was in sinus rhythm, with a normal volume pulse. The venous pressure was normal, but a dominant 'a' wave was noted. The apex beat was sustained. On auscultation there was a long, grade 3 out of 4, systolic murmur that was maximal down the left sternal edge. The peripheral pulses were present and equal. The remainder of the physical examination revealed no abnormality.

Screening test results

Haemoglobin	13.9 g/dl	ESR	3 mm/1st hr
WBC	6.1×10^9/l	MCV	84 fl
Potassium	3.8 mmol/l	Sodium	139 mmol/l
Bicarbonate	25 mmol/l	Chloride	104 mmol/l
Urea	4.7 mmol/l	Creatinine	67 μmol/l
Calcium	2.46 mmol/l	Phosphate	1.05 mmol/l
Total Protein	68 g/l	Albumin	41 g/l
Bilirubin	5 μmol/l		
Aspartate		Alkaline	
Transaminase	14 U/l	Phosphatase	44 U/l

Urine analysis: normal

The Viva: questions and answers on page 123.

Recurrent chest infections

A 59-year-old labourer, with a five-year history of chronic lymphocytic leukaemia, came to the haematology clinic complaining that he felt very ill. He was feverish and was coughing up large quantities of green sputum; he had a poor appetite and had lost 10 kg over the past six months. During that time he had repeated courses of antibiotics for recurrent minor chest infections. Six years earlier he had presented with glandular enlargement at many sites and splenomegaly. Several courses of treatment with allopurinol, chlorambucil and prednisolone had led to reduction of lymph node size and splenomegaly.

On examination he looked haggard, flushed and had obviously lost weight. His temperature was 40°C, pulse 112/min. There was dullness and bronchial breathing at the left base, with bilateral crepitations. Enlarged lymph nodes were present in both axillae and groins; the spleen was palpable 7 cm below the costal margin. Numerous petechial haemorrhages and bruises were present on his arms and legs.

Screening test results

Haemoglobin	9.8 g/dl	ESR	11 mm/1st hr
WBC	47.8 × 10⁹/l	MCV	86 fl
Potassium	4.5 mmol/l	Sodium	128 mmol/l
Bicarbonate	23 mmol/l	Chloride	99 mmol/l
Urea	4.1 mmol/l	Creatinine	103 μmol/l
Calcium	2.26 mmol/l	Phosphate	0.92 mmol/l
Total Protein	50 g/l	Albumin	33 g/l
Bilirubin	14 μmol/l		
Aspartate		Alkaline	
Transaminase	37 U/l	Phosphatase	123 U/l

Urine analysis: normal

The Viva: questions and answers on page 158.

Failed medical check-up

A 35-year-old single businessman presented for a routine medical check-up. He had felt slightly tired after a long day's work but was otherwise well. He denied excessive intake of alcohol, recent foreign travel, a past history of hepatitis, regular intake of any medication, or contact with a patient suffering from hepatitis.

Examination showed a well-developed, healthy-looking man. An enlarged liver was felt below the right costal margin. The edge was firm and non-tender. The spleen was not palpable, but the splenic area was dull to percussion. There was no peripheral oedema and no other abnormal physical sign.

Screening test results

Haemoglobin	15.0 g/dl	ESR	20 mm/1st hr
WBC	5.0 × 10⁹/l	MCV	85 fl
Potassium	4.3 mmol/l	Sodium	138 mmol/l
Bicarbonate	24 mmol/l	Chloride	102 mmol/l
Urea	3.4 mmol/l	Creatinine	76 μmol/l
Calcium	2.49 mmol/l	Phosphate	1.01 mmol/l
Total Protein	79 g/l	Albumin	42 g/l
Bilirubin	34 μmol/l		
Aspartate		Alkaline	
Transaminase	160 U/l	Phosphatase	90 U/l

Urine analysis: urobilinogen + + ; bilirubin −

The Viva: questions and answers on page 236.

Academic decline

A 57-year-old male university lecturer presented with a 12-month history of memory impairment and poor concentration. He complained that he found it increasingly difficult to cope with his teaching responsibilities and he doubted whether his previous academic publications had been of much value. Some of his colleagues had recently been offered early retirement and he feared that he would be made redundant as part of his university's financial savings. On direct questioning he admitted to lowering of mood with diurnal variation, early morning wakening, loss of appetite and declining libido. On physical examination he looked unkempt and showed evidence of motor and mental retardation. There were signs of recent weight loss but otherwise the examination was normal.

Screening test results

Haemoglobin	14.5 g/dl	ESR	5 mm/1st hr
WBC	$6.2 \times 10^9/l$	MCV	91 fl
Potassium	3.9 mmol/l	Sodium	139 mmol/l
Bicarbonate	26 mmol/l	Chloride	98 mmol/l
Urea	4.2 mmol/l	Creatinine	92 μmol/l
Calcium	2.42 mmol/l	Phosphate	0.75 mmol/l
Total Protein	72 g/l	Albumin	48 g/l
Bilirubin	7 μmol/l		
Aspartate		Alkaline	
Transaminase	12 U/l	Phosphatase	38 U/l

Urine analysis: normal

The Viva: questions and answers on page 100.

Weight loss and stiffness

A widow aged 72 complained of malaise, poor appetite and weight loss. These symptoms had developed fairly rapidly during a three-week period: her weight had dropped from 68 to 64 kg. Six months earlier her husband had died after a long illness, and her family had noticed that she was finding it very difficult to cope alone. She had become extremely stiff and complained of pains in the muscles across her neck and shoulders. She had had no headaches or scalp tenderness, and her vision was normal. She found it difficult to get up in the mornings and her daughter had been visiting every day to help her to dress.

On examination she was thin and depressed; she appeared anaemic. There were no enlarged lymph nodes, and no masses were found in her breasts or thyroid. Her temporal arteries were normal. Her muscles were not tender and there was no proximal weakness. Shoulder movements were painful and reduced in all directions. No arterial bruits were heard and her fundi were normal. No other abnormalities were found in the rest of the physical examination.

Screening test results

Haemoglobin	10.4 g/dl	ESR	96 mm/1st hr
WBC	6.2×10^9/l	MCV	84 fl
Potassium	4.4 mmol/l	Sodium	138 mmol/l
Bicarbonate	24 mmol/l	Chloride	102 mmol/l
Urea	9.2 mmol/l	Creatinine	130 μmol/l
Calcium	2.43 mmol/l	Phosphate	1.17 mmol/l
Total Protein	70 g/l	Albumin	37 g/l
Bilirubin	8 μmol/l		
Aspartate		Alkaline	
Transaminase	29 U/l	Phosphatase	140 U/l

Urine analysis: normal

The Viva: questions and answers on page 197.

A fat boy

An 18-year-old petrol attendant was referred to the clinic with obesity; he had no other complaint. He had been a full-term normal delivery, and until the age of 13 had achieved all the normal milestones. About that time it was noticed that he was smaller than his class-mates. He was of normal intelligence, but had gradually become rather slow and apathetic.

Examination revealed a very shy, obese boy with no evidence of a beard, absence of pubic and axillary hair, a small penis and testicles, and absent rugosity of his scrotum. His height was less than expected when compared with the size of his parents and siblings.

His visual fields and fundi were normal, there was no limb weakness, but his reflexes showed a slow relaxation phase. The breasts were rather prominent, and a minimal amount of serous secretion could be expressed from the left nipple.

Screening test results

Haemoglobin	15.0 g/dl	ESR	8 mm/1st hr
WBC	5.7×10^9/l	MCV	94 fl
Potassium	5.1 mmol/l	Sodium	136 mmol/l
Bicarbonate	21 mmol/l	Chloride	98 mmol/l
Urea	3.8 mmol/l	Creatinine	67 μmol/l
Calcium	2.56 mmol/l	Phosphate	1.15 mmol/l
Total Protein	75 g/l	Albumin	46 g/l
Bilirubin	5 μmol/l		
Aspartate		Alkaline	
Transaminase	28 U/l	Phosphatase	72 U/l

Urine analysis: normal

The Viva: questions and answers on page 72.

A lump in the neck

A 33-year-old male porter presented complaining of a lump in the neck, chest pain and feeling unwell. His symptoms had started two weeks before with a flu-like illness. In the week before admission, sharp central chest pains developed whilst he was out drinking in a pub, and they lasted about 30 minutes. The pain radiated through to his back and was felt also in the lumbar region. He felt a tender lump in the right side of his neck and came straight up to casualty. He had a sore throat at the start of the illness and had also noticed some night sweats. Previously, he had enjoyed good health and he had not lost weight.

On examination, he was slightly febrile (37.7°C) and looked unwell, but was not jaundiced. There were two hard, tender lymph nodes in the right supraclavicular fossa, each about 1 cm in diameter. His tonsils were not enlarged. Examination of his cardiovascular, respiratory and central nervous systems was normal. His liver was not palpable, but the spleen could be felt quite easily.

Screening test results

Haemoglobin	15.0 g/dl	ESR	13 mm/1st hr
WBC	10.1 × 10^9/l	MCV	87 fl
Potassium	4.4 mmol/l	Sodium	139 mmol/l
Bicarbonate	27 mmol/l	Chloride	102 mmol/l
Urea	3.6 mmol/l	Creatinine	92 μmol/l
Calcium	2.47 mmol/l	Phosphate	1.01 mmol/l
Total Protein	68 g/l	Albumin	40 g/l
Bilirubin	12 μmol/l		
Aspartate		Alkaline	
Transaminase	36 U/l	Phosphatase	54 U/l

Urine analysis: normal

The Viva: questions and answers on page 128.

A bearded lady

A 21-year-old female shop assistant presented with a history of excessive facial hair for a year, and amenorrhoea for six months. Over the last year, she had gained 5 kg in weight, had felt depressed and had noticed diminished libido. Three years earlier she had started the contraceptive pill, which she had stopped six months prior to her presentation.

On examination she was overweight but normotensive. The facial hair was thick and excessive, as was the hair on her limbs. She had a normal skin, with no acne. Her voice was soft and feminine. Abdominal examination revealed no masses, and vaginal examination was also normal. The external genitalia were of normal size.

Screening test results

Haemoglobin	12.5 g/dl	ESR	4 mm/1st hr
WBC	8.3 × 10⁹/l	MCV	86 fl
Potassium	4.6 mmol/l	Sodium	139 mmol/l
Bicarbonate	24 mmol/l	Chloride	100 mmol/l
Urea	4.3 mmol/l	Creatinine	62 µmol/l
Calcium	2.34 mmol/l	Phosphate	1.12 mmol/l
Total Protein	70 g/l	Albumin	42 g/l
Bilirubin	11 µmol/l		
Aspartate		Alkaline	
Transaminase	25 U/l	Phosphatase	72 U/l

Urine analysis: normal

The Viva: questions and answers on page 184.

Increasing malaise

For the past nine months a 57-year-old carpenter had not felt really well. He had struggled to work, but was becoming increasingly tired and found it difficult to concentrate for a full day. He noticed some swelling of the ankles in the evening, and his gums and nose bled slightly in the mornings. His appetite was poor. His urine was dark in the mornings, but the stools were a normal colour.

Four weeks previously he had suffered influenza with the rest of his family, but afterwards he found his abdomen increasing in size so that he could not do up his trousers. His weight had increased. He slept poorly and sometimes had difficulty in holding a cup in the morning. His wife noticed his breath was occasionally unpleasant. He denied excessive consumption of alcohol, he had never suffered from hepatitis and he took no regular drugs. There was no family history of liver disease. He ate a good diet. He had never received a blood transfusion.

On examination he weighed 80 kg (his usual weight was 70 kg). His temperature was 37°C. His complexion was muddy. His eyes were slightly yellow and his cheeks sunken. The tongue was dry and furred, and fetor hepaticus was present. Small vascular spiders were seen on the face, necklace area, shoulders and hands. The palms were red and mottled. There was a coarse tremor of the outstretched hands. He had difficulty in remembering recent events and in performing mental arithmetic. The JVP was raised 4 cm above the sternal angle. His blood pressure was 100/70. The circulation was hyperdynamic with an apical systolic murmur also heard in the axilla. In contrast to a very distended abdomen, the limbs were spindly with a 'spider man' appearance due to muscle wasting. The abdominal distension was particularly in the flanks, the umbilicus being everted. The skin was shiny. Distended abdominal veins were seen around the umbilicus, the direction of flow being away from the navel. Shifting dullness could be detected and there was a fluid thrill. The viscera were difficult to palpate, but a firm liver edge could be felt 8 cm below the left costal margin and, on 'dipping', the spleen was also probably felt 4 cm below the left costal margin; the splenic area was dull to percussion. There was no abdominal tenderness. Tendon reflexes were brisk and the plantar responses flexor. Pitting oedema of the ankles was present. Sexual hair was scanty and the testes were small and soft.

Screening test results

Haemoglobin	10.3 g/dl	ESR	40 mm/1st hr
WBC	3.2×10^9/l	MCV	88 fl
Potassium	4.3 mmol/l	Sodium	132 mmol/l
Bicarbonate	27 mmol/l	Chloride	98 mmol/l
Urea	3.0 mmol/l	Creatinine	86 μmol/l
Calcium	2.37 mmol/l	Phosphate	1.15 mmol/l
Total Protein	78 g/l	Albumin	28 g/l
Bilirubin	50 μmol/l		
Aspartate		Alkaline	
Transaminase	120 U/l	Phosphatase	180 U/l

Urine analysis: urobilinogen + + +; bilirubin trace

The Viva: questions and answers on page 175.

Cold fingers

A secretary aged 50 complained that her fingertips had become so painful that she could no longer type. Since childhood her fingers had blanched on exposure to cold and she described the typical colour changes of Raynaud's phenomenon. During the year prior to presentation her fingers had remained persistently cold and purplish in colour, and had become swollen. Painful ulcers had developed on the tips of several fingers.

Her only other complaint was of heartburn; she attributed occasional slight difficulty in swallowing food to this. She had found that sleeping propped-up by several pillows alleviated the heartburn.

On examination she appeared well. The skin of her fingers was cyanosed and there was subcutaneous swelling. There was pulp atrophy and terminal pitting ulceration of several fingers. The skin on the dorsum of her hands seemed thickened, although the patient had noticed no change. Her facial appearance was normal, as was the remainder of the physical examination. Her blood pressure was 130/70.

Screening test results

Haemoglobin	12.8 g/dl	ESR	30 mm/1st hr
WBC	5.6 × 10^9/l	MCV	83 fl
Potassium	4.6 mmol/l	Sodium	139 mmol/l
Bicarbonate	26 mmol/l	Chloride	104 mmol/l
Urea	4.2 mmol/l	Creatinine	72 μmol/l
Calcium	2.47 mmol/l	Phosphate	1.07 mmol/l
Total Protein	78 g/l	Albumin	40 g/l
Bilirubin	10 μmol/l		
Aspartate		Alkaline	
Transaminase	24 U/l	Phosphatase	39 U/l

Urine analysis: normal

The Viva: questions and answers on page 106.

Continuing dyspepsia

A 56-year-old printer presented with unremitting epigastric pain seven months after emergency gastric surgery. He described several years of uninvestigated dyspepsia which finally resulted in an emergency hospital admission due to haematemesis and melaena. The patient continued to bleed, so after 24 hours he had an emergency laparotomy. The patient reported that the surgeon had found a big ulcer that penetrated the pancreas. The patient did not know whether the ulcer was in the stomach or duodenum, nor the exact surgical procedure.

After the operation, the haemorrhage stopped and the patient made a rapid recovery. However, he soon developed progressively severe epigastric pain. He had never been well enough to return to work after the operation. The pain was unrelieved by cimetidine or antispasmodics. As the pain became progressively more severe, the patient started to vomit and he lost 7 kg. He was sleeping badly and felt generally unwell.

On examination the patient was pale and had recently lost weight. There was no abnormality in the cardiovascular, respiratory or alimentary systems, apart from epigastric tenderness.

Screening test results

Haemoglobin	8.4 g/dl	ESR	34 mm/1st hr
WBC	$5.6 \times 10^9/l$	MCV	77 fl
Potassium	3.4 mmol/l	Sodium	139 mmol/l
Bicarbonate	25 mmol/l	Chloride	104 mmol/l
Urea	5.9 mmol/l	Creatinine	76 μmol/l
Calcium	2.45 mmol/l	Phosphate	1.05 mmol/l
Total Protein	68 g/l	Albumin	41 g/l
Bilirubin	5 μmol/l		
Aspartate		Alkaline	
Transaminase	14 U/l	Phosphatase	44 U/l

Urine analysis: normal

The Viva: questions and answers on page 193.

Oliguria after multiple injuries

An 18-year-old unemployed man sustained extensive injuries to both legs following a motorcycle accident. Both his legs were trapped underneath a car for two hours before he was freed and transferred to hospital.

On examination he was shocked: he was hypotensive with a blood pressure of 60/40 and a pulse rate of 130/min. His left leg was extensively bruised, tense and swollen. Peripheral pulses could not be felt below the femoral artery on the left. The right leg was less swollen but there was a compound fracture of the right tibia and fibula, with extensive damage and contamination of the muscles of the anterior tibial compartment. In the casualty department a drip was set up and he was given two litres of normal saline which restored his blood pressure to 110/70. His compound fracture was treated with surgical debridement and internal fixation was carried out. Post-operatively he was given 80 mg of gentamicin eight-hourly and 500 mg of flucloxacillin six-hourly. 24 hours after admission it was noticed that he had only passed 50 ml of dark brown urine.

Screening test results

Haemoglobin	11.4 g/dl	ESR	64 mm/1st hr
WBC	17.4×10^9/l	MCV	89 fl
Potassium	7.1 mmol/l	Sodium	143 mmol/l
Bicarbonate	11 mmol/l	Chloride	98 mmol/l
Urea	24.3 mmol/l	Creatinine	831 μmol/l
Calcium	1.22 mmol/l	Phosphate	3.2 mmol/l
Total Protein	60 g/l	Albumin	28 g/l
Bilirubin	25 μmol/l		
Aspartate Transaminase	300 U/l	Alkaline Phosphatase	128 U/l

Urine analysis: blood + +; protein +

The Viva: questions and answers on page 209.

A Chelsea pensioner

A 68-year-old Chelsea pensioner blamed his respiratory distress to the fact that he was gassed in the First World War, although he was only born during that war! This explanation blinded him to the fact that he was a heavy smoker, living and working in the polluted atmosphere of Battersea all his life. For many years he had suffered from cough and phlegm, not only in winter but also through the summer months. He was admitted to hospital as an emergency, as he had become suddenly weaker and more short of breath.

On examination he was centrally cyanosed, obese and barrel-chested. He produced large amounts of yellow sputum. There were engorged neck veins, warm extremities, and pulmonary added sounds; the liver was enlarged and oedema spread from his legs to the sacrum. He had a bounding pulse and flapping tremor. He was extremely short of breath at rest, showing pursed-lip expiration. He had a flame-shaped subconjunctival haemorrhage in the right eye and papilloedema in both eyes.

Screening test results

Haemoglobin	17.7 g/dl	ESR	32 mm/1st hr
WBC	15.1×10^9/l	MCV	84 fl
Potassium	3.9 mmol/l	Sodium	137 mmol/l
Bicarbonate	31 mmol/l	Chloride	102 mmol/l
Urea	9.8 mmol/l	Creatinine	98 μmol/l
Calcium	2.52 mmol/l	Phosphate	1.02 mmol/l
Total Protein	79 g/l	Albumin	35 g/l
Bilirubin	16 μmol/l		
Aspartate		Alkaline	
Transaminase	67 U/l	Phosphatase	172 U/l

Urine analysis: albumin + only

The Viva: questions and answers on page 166.

Haematuria

A 51-year-old farmer was transferred to the teaching hospital because of bruising and haematuria. 10 months previously, whilst on holiday in Morocco, he had haematuria and haematospermia; an *E.coli* urinary tract infection was found which cleared up with antibiotics. Four months later he again developed haematuria, but there was no infection. His prostate was hard; an IVP was normal but the X-ray did show calcification in the prostate; cytoscopy was normal but a prostatic biopsy did not confirm the clinical diagnosis of prostatic carcinoma. The plasma acid phosphatase was normal.

The patient was admitted to hospital as the haematuria had recurred, but it was much heavier. In addition, he had developed extensive bruising over his right leg, on his hands and on his chest. Also he complained of pain in the right side of his jaw, and of lower abdominal pain and distension which had developed over the preceding two days.

A blood transfusion was already in progress when the patient arrived at the teaching hospital. On examination there was extensive bruising on the right side of his neck, on his legs and around the umbilicus. There were blood blisters present on the soft palate. A urinary catheter was in place, and the urine was heavily bloodstained. Bruising was present around venepuncture sites.

Screening test results

Haemoglobin	7.5 g/dl	ESR	12 mm/1st hr
WBC	13.6×10^9/l	MCV	90 fl
Potassium	4.2 mmol/l	Sodium	136 mmol/l
Bicarbonate	27 mmol/l	Chloride	102 mmol/l
Urea	7.2 mmol/l	Creatinine	112 μmol/l
Calcium	2.24 mmol/l	Phosphate	1.23 mmol/l
Total Protein	60 g/l	Albumin	34 g/l
Bilirubin	23 μmol/l		
Aspartate Transaminase	38 U/l	Alkaline Phosphatase	36 U/l

Urine analysis: protein + +; white cells +; red cells + + + +

The Viva: questions and answers on page 242.

Confusion in an alcoholic

A 48-year-old man who lived alone was brought to hospital by the police having been found collapsed on the pavement outside his home. He was well-known as being a heavy drinker, but he had appeared well when seen by neighbours the previous day. He had not worked for several years and spent most of his unemployment benefit on beer, tending to drink with acquaintances at a local public house.

On examination the patient was thin and his breath smelt slightly of alcohol. He was drowsy, ataxic and his speech was slurred. There were lateral rectus palsies, a horizontal nystagmus, sluggish tendon reflexes and reduced sensation to pinprick and light touch. He was disorientated in time and place, and he could not give a coherent account of his recent activities. The only other abnormal sign was that his liver was palpable 3 cm below the right costal margin.

Screening test results

Haemoglobin	13.5 g/dl	ESR	6 mm/1st hr
WBC	6.2 × 10⁹/l	MCV	108 fl
Potassium	3.9 mmol/l	Sodium	142 mmol/l
Bicarbonate	23 mmol/l	Chloride	102 mmol/l
Urea	4.9 mmol/l	Creatinine	69 μmol/1
Calcium	2.21 mmol/l	Phosphate	1.08 mmol/l
Total Protein	62 g/l	Albumim	33 g/l
Bilirubin	7 μmol/l		
Aspartate		Alkaline	
Transaminase	73 U/l	Phosphatase	69 U/l

Urine analysis: normal

The Viva: questions and answers on page 169.

25

Progressive weakness

A 22-year-old medical student complained of malaise and back pain made worse by movement. He had had a non-specific febrile illness one week previously. The following day he noticed difficulty in walking with a tendency to foot-drop. This progressed rapidly over three days to severe weakness of the legs and arms, with some difficulty in swallowing and nasal regurgitation of fluids. No loss of feeling was noticed, but he had paraesthesiae in hands and feet. He developed retention of urine.

On examination he was mentally alert but anxious. Ocular movements were full. There was bilateral facial weakness and the palate moved poorly. The cough was weak. There was flaccid weakness of all limbs and trunk, with absent tendon reflexes. Plantar responses were unobtainable. There was no sensory loss.

Screening test results

Haemoglobin	15.4 g/dl	ESR	12 mm/1st hr
WBC	6.0 × 10⁹/l	MCV	86 fl
Potassium	3.8 mmol/l	Sodium	138 mmol/l
Bicarbonate	24 mmol/l	Chloride	96 mmol/l
Urea	4.5 mmol/l	Creatinine	104 μmol/l
Calcium	2.41 mmol/l	Phosphate	0.75 mmol/l
Total Protein	68 g/l	Albumin	46 g/l
Bilirubin	5 μmol/l		
Aspartate		Alkaline	
Transaminase	10 U/l	Phosphatase	35 U/l

Urine analysis: normal

The Viva: questions and answers on page 200.

A young stroke

A 26-year-old housewife was admitted for investigation of an episode of numbness and weakness of the left arm. This had occurred suddenly two days earlier, and had almost completely resolved by the time of admission. There had been no difficulty with speech, although the patient had noted a left-sided facial weakness. Fine movements of the left hand remained impaired. Six months previously, she had been admitted to a surgical ward with pain in the left upper quadrant of the abdomen, accompanied by tenderness and nausea, but no vomiting. However, her symptoms subsided spontaneously and she was discharged without any definite diagnosis. The patient was married, with two children, aged five and three, and was taking a low-oestrogen oral contraceptive pill.

On examination, she was right-handed. In the central nervous system the only abnormal physical sign was a slight increase in the tendon jerks of the left arm. The cranial nerves were intact, the fundi normal, and both plantars flexor. There was no cyanosis or clubbing of the fingers. The venous pressure was normal. A late systolic murmur was noted on admission, but this was not confirmed at a subsequent ward round. There was no femoral delay, but the right anterior tibial pulse was absent. The blood pressure was 110/70. The chest was clear and the abdomen normal to palpation. Homan's sign was negative.

Screening test results

Haemoglobin	10.5 g/dl	ESR	85 mm/1st hr
WBC	7.6×10^9/l	MCV	85 fl
Potassium	4.2 mmol/l	Sodium	137 mmol/l
Bicarbonate	27 mmol/l	Chloride	102 mmol/l
Urea	5.0 mmol/l	Creatinine	89 μmol/l
Calcium	2.34 mmol/l	Phosphate	0.84 mmol/l
Total Protein	85 g/l	Albumin	41 g/l
Bilirubin	20 μmol/l		
Aspartate		Alkaline	
Transaminase	25 U/l	Phosphatase	75 U/l

Urine analysis: normal

The Viva: questions and answers on page 98.

Pruritus for six months

A 48-year-old English married housewife presented with a six-month history of itching. This started gradually, but was now bad, particularly at night when she was warm in bed. She had noticed darkening of the skin over the last two to three years. She also complained of morning stiffness of the fingers. Her eyes tended to be dry and tears did not come easily. Her mouth was also dry. The urine was occasionally dark in the morning. Her weight was steady, her appetite good, and she felt well in herself.

15 years before she had had a partial thyroidectomy for a goitre. She did not take any medications. She had never taken oral contraceptives or hormones. She had never suffered from colitis or diarrhoea. In the family, one sister gave a history of arthritis and another of swelling of the neck. There was no family history of liver disease. She had two children who were well and had left home. Her husband was a butcher.

On examination the patient appeared well. The skin was pigmented, particularly on exposed parts. She was not jaundiced; there were no xanthelasmata. She was clinically euthyroid and the thyroid was not palpable. There was some enlargement of the proximal interphalangeal joints, and the skin was slightly thickened over the fingers. The liver was enlarged 6 cm below the costal margin on deep inspiration. The edge was firm, smooth and non-tender. The spleen was easily palpable 5 cm below the left costal margin. There was no ascites or oedema.

Screening test results

Haemoglobin	12.3 g/dl	ESR	35 mm/1st hr
WBC	6.8 × 10⁹/l	MCV	86 fl
Potassium	4.0 mmol/l	Sodium	139 mmol/l
Bicarbonate	28 mmol/l	Chloride	103 mmol/l
Urea	4.4 mmol/l	Creatinine	66 μmol/l
Calcium	2.31 mmol/l	Phosphate	1.13 mmol/l
Total Protein	80 g/l	Albumin	39 g/l
Bilirubin	12 μmol/l		
Aspartate		Alkaline	
Transaminase	63 U/l	Phosphatase	204 U/l

Urine analysis: urobilinogen + + + +; bilirubin −

The Viva: questions and answers on page 155.

Backache

A lawyer aged 26 complained of low backache. The pain was mainly troublesome at night and he found his back to be particularly stiff for the first hour after waking. The backache had developed gradually over the preceding year, and was partly relieved by aspirin tablets. He was a keen squash player but intermittently found that left heel pain, lasting for up to three weeks, made it impossible for him to play.

Five years previously he had been seen by an ophthalmologist for an acutely painful red eye. Iritis was diagnosed which responded to a short course of mydriatic and steroid eye drops.

He denied any rash, bowel or urinary symptoms. However, he recalled that a cousin had ulcerative colitis and that his father had psoriasis.

On examination he was fit and athletic in appearance. His lumbar spine was stiff in all movements, and lateral flexion and extension of his lumbar spine was particularly limited. Forward flexion of his lumbar spine was limited to 3 cm. On attempting to touch his toes without flexing his knees he could only reach 20 cm from the ground. Chest expansion was reduced to 3 cm. Pressure over his sacro-iliac joints and ischial tuberosities caused considerable pain. His left heel was tender to pressure. Both eyes were normal.

The remainder of the examination was normal, in particular, there were no abnormal cardiovascular signs or cardiac murmurs.

Screening test results

Haemoglobin	14.6 g/dl	ESR	12 mm/1st hr
WBC	4.9×10^9/l	MCV	80 fl
Potassium	4.2 mmol/l	Sodium	136 mmol/l
Bicarbonate	22 mmol/l	Chloride	100 mmol/l
Urea	4.1 mmol/l	Creatinine	96 μmol/l
Calcium	2.34 mmol/l	Phosphate	1.06 mmol/l
Total Protein	76 g/l	Albumin	48 g/l
Bilirubin	6 μmol/l		
Aspartate		Alkaline	
Transaminase	24 U/l	Phosphatase	42 U/l

Urine analysis: normal

The Viva: questions and answers on page 217.

Bloody diarrhoea

A 59-year-old single building labourer had enjoyed good health until two years ago, when he noticed occasional bouts of diarrhoea. A barium enema showed diverticular disease of the sigmoid colon. His symptoms settled spontaneously and he felt better after starting a high fibre diet.

Approximately one month before presentation, he became unwell. He developed diarrhoea, low abdominal pain, and within days blood in the stools. His family doctor diagnosed a further attack of diverticulitis and prescribed ampicillin. The patient's health declined rapidly with continuing bloody diarrhoea, fever, anorexia and loss of weight.

He was admitted as an emergency. He was ill, pale, febrile and had oral candida. He had red eyes, but neither arthritis nor a skin rash. Examination revealed a slightly distended abdomen with no sign of peritonitis. The anus was healthy, but the surrounding skin excoriated.

Screening test results

Haemoglobin	8.2 g/dl	ESR	80 mm/1st hr
WBC	4.9×10^9/l	MCV	77 fl
Potassium	4.8 mmol/l	Sodium	128 mmol/l
Bicarbonate	23 mmol/l	Chloride	94 mmol/l
Urea	2.0 mmol/l	Creatinine	58 μmol/l
Calcium	2.11 mmol/l	Phosphate	1.00 mmol/l
Total Protein	58 g/l	Albumin	24 g/l
Bilirubin	6 μmol/l		
Aspartate		Alkaline	
Transaminase	34 U/l	Phosphatase	102 U/l

Urine analysis: normal

The Viva: questions and answers on page 80.

A multisystem disease?

A 19-year-old student went to the accident and emergency department with a short history of general ill health, backache and joint pains. For two days he had noticed that he was only passing small volumes of dark urine. Two weeks before he had developed a cold, with a cough and sore throat which lasted five days. He was given penicillin by his general practitioner but he stopped it after six days because he developed a generalised maculo-papular rash on his abdomen, trunk and arms.

On examination he had a trace of ankle oedema. He was apyrexial and there was no lymphadenopathy. The JVP was raised 2 cm. The blood pressure was 190/105. Examination of the chest and abdomen was unremarkable. The fundi showed occasional haemorrhages and exudates, but no papilloedema. A neurological examination was normal.

Screening test results

Haemoglobin	14.3 g/dl	ESR	68 mm/1st hr
WBC	9.3×10^9/l	MCV	84 fl
Potassium	5.3 mmol/l	Sodium	129 mmol/l
Bicarbonate	21 mmol/l	Chloride	93 mmol/l
Urea	28.6 mmol/l	Creatinine	238 μmol/l
Calcium	2.27 mmol/l	Phosphate	1.89 mmol/l
Total Protein	67 g/l	Albumin	30 g/l
Bilirubin	4 μmol/l		
Aspartate		Alkaline	
Transaminase	29 U/l	Phosphatase	85 U/l

Urine analysis: blood + + + ; protein + +

The Viva: questions and answers on page 134.

Tachypnoea

A 17-year-old college student developed vague right chest pain with associated hyperventilation. Within 12 hours of the start of symptoms, she was seen by her doctor who attributed it to anxiety, since the father had recently died of bronchial carcinoma and the impressionable daughter was anxiously endeavouring to give up smoking. Her vague complaints came to a head when the right chest pain became clearly pleuritic and was associated with severe breathlessness.

When the family doctor re-examined her, she was not only very anxious but also distressed and in obvious pain. This restricted her breathing to a shallow tachypnoea, which was associated with a friction rub. Whilst the doctor was still deciding whether to send her for an out-patient chest X-ray or to arrange a specialist domiciliary consultation, she had a haemoptysis. This frightened her and also the doctor, who then arranged her immediate hospital admission.

On admission, the patient was scared but not shocked. She was not cyanosed but had a temperature of 37.8°C. She had a pulse of 120/min in sinus rhythm, with a blood pressure of 100/70. The JVP was not elevated, and the heart sounds were normal. There was no peripheral oedema, nor calf tenderness.

Screening test results

Haemoglobin	12.3 g/dl	ESR	27 mm/1st hr
WBC	$10.7 \times 10^9/l$	MCV	83 fl
Potassium	4.3 mmol/l	Sodium	140 mmol/l
Bicarbonate	21 mmol/l	Chloride	95 mmol/l
Urea	3.7 mmol/l	Creatinine	72 μmol/l
Calcium	2.22 mmol/l	Phosphate	1.13 mmol/l
Total Protein	76 g/l	Albumin	45 g/l
Bilirubin	8 μmol/l		
Aspartate		Alkaline	
Transaminase	31 U/l	Phosphatase	53 U/l

Urine analysis: normal

The Viva: questions and answers on page 66.

Heart failure

A 70-year-old woman was admitted with a two-month history of breathlessness on exertion. For one week before admission she had been woken by retrosternal pain and breathlessness, which had responded to sublingual glyceryl trinitrate. Exercise tolerance was limited, by breathlessness and chest pain, to walking for about 400 yards slowly on the level. She had nocturia for one month, and for two weeks she had a dry cough. She smoked 20 cigarettes a day for many years, and for 10 years had mild diabetes, controlled by diet alone.

Six months previously she had had a full-thickness anterior myocardial infarction, complicated by three attacks of ventricular fibrillation from which she had been successfully resuscitated. She had been given intravenous lignocaine, followed by mexilitene for one month. The latter drug was stopped as she developed extrapyramidal side effects. A 24-hour tape at this time had shown ventricular ectopic beats only.

On examination, she was orthopnoeic. She was in sinus rhythm at a rate of 100/min. The blood pressure was 140/90, and the venous pressure was raised 5 cm, with a dominant 'v' wave. An abnormal right parasternal impulse was palpable and the apex beat was sustained. On auscultation, there was a soft pansystolic murmur and a third heart sound at the apex. Pulmonary valve closure was accentuated. There were crepitations at the lung bases. The liver was enlarged 4 cm below the right costal margin.

Screening test results

Haemoglobin	13.9 g/dl	ESR	12 mm/1st hr
WBC	5.1×10^9/l	MCV	85 fl
Potassium	3.5 mmol/l	Sodium	130 mmol/l
Bicarbonate	29 mmol/l	Chloride	100 mmol/l
Urea	8.0 mmol/l	Creatinine	121 μmol/l
Calcium	2.40 mmol/l	Phosphate	0.89 mmol/l
Total Protein	75 g/l	Albumin	41 g/l
Bilirubin	12 μmol/l		
Aspartate		Alkaline	
Transaminase	33 U/l	Phosphatase	79 U/l

Urine analysis: normal

The Viva: questions and answers on page 109.

Sickle cell anaemia

A 17-year-old Jamaican-born girl shop assistant with sickle cell anaemia attended the casualty department because of pain in her back and legs. Since coming to England, she had been admitted to hospital on numerous occasions for episodes of abdominal and bone pain, as well as for infective crises. She attended the outpatient department on a fairly regular basis and was maintained on folic acid 5 mg daily. Five days before this admission, she woke up with a frontal headache, sore throat and fever. Three days later she consulted her doctor who prescribed ampicillin. Later that day, pain started in her back and legs. In addition, she became increasingly short of breath and she felt shivery.

On examination she looked unwell but was not pyrexial. She appeared anaemic but was not jaundiced. Apart from some tenderness over the sacrum and around the malleoli, no abnormality was detected during full examination.

She was admitted for observation with the provisional diagnosis of a sickle cell crisis, and given analgesics and intravenous fluids (3 litres a day). Next morning she had a mild pyrexia with no localising signs; she was put on amoxycillin 250 mg tds. Later that day, she became acutely ill with severe dyspnoea, tachypnoea (respiration rate 50/min), tachycardia (130/min) and a pyrexia of 40.5 °C. Dullness, poor air entry and coarse crepitations were detected on the right side of her chest. She was transferred to the intensive care unit.

Screening test results

Haemoglobin	4.0 g/dl	ESR	76 mm/1st hr
WBC	14.6 × 10⁹/l	MCV	83 fl
Potassium	3.2 mmol/l	Sodium	130 mmol/l
Bicarbonate	19 mmol/l	Chloride	95 mmol/l
Urea	4.3 mmol/l	Creatinine	104 μmol/l
Calcium	2.21 mmol/l	Phosphate	1.13 mmol/l
Total Protein	69 g/l	Albumin	40 g/l
Bilirubin	16 μmol/l		
Aspartate		Alkaline	
Transaminase	38 U/l	Phosphatase	102 U/l

Urine analysis: red cells only

The Viva: questions and answers on page 83.

A little stroke

An electrician of 55 experienced a sudden onset of clumsiness and paraesthesiae in the left hand and arm whilst cleaning his car. At the same time he noticed numbness and stiffness of the left side of the face and tongue. The symptoms resolved completely within 10 minutes. Over the next month three further attacks occurred, each with complete recovery. There was a past history of mild myocardial infarction two years before. He had had two attacks of brief visual loss in the right eye in the past six months. He smoked 20 cigarettes per day.

On examination there were no abnormal signs in the central nervous system. In the cardiovascular system the heart sounds were normal; the pulse was 80/min in sinus rhythm. A systolic bruit was heard on both sides of the neck. The superficial temporal pulse was delayed on the left. Both radial pulses were synchronous, and the blood pressure was 160/100 in each arm.

Screening test results

Haemoglobin	17.0 g/dl	ESR	2 mm/1st hr
WBC	9.0×10^9/l	MCV	84 fl
Potassium	4.0 mmol/l	Sodium	145 mmol/l
Bicarbonate	26 mmol/l	Chloride	100 mmol/l
Urea	5.0 mmol/l	Creatinine	104 μmol/l
Calcium	2.40 mmol/l	Phosphate	0.80 mmol/l
Total Protein	76 g/l	Albumin	40 g/l
Bilirubin	5 μmol/l		
Aspartate		Alkaline	
Transaminase	20 U/l	Phosphatase	44 U/l

Urine analysis: normal

The Viva: questions and answers on page 239.

Over-activity following childbirth

A 26-year-old woman was brought to the Accident and Emergency Department by her husband. He reported that she had given birth to their first child two weeks previously and had been discharged from hospital after 48 hours. Two days later he became concerned that she was more restless and irritable than usual. She became progressively more over-active, slept for only two or three hours each night and ignored her baby's crying — even though she considered it to be especially gifted. She had spent the equivalent of two months of her husband's salary on clothes during the previous week and, on her way home from a shopping expedition, had been involved in a minor car crash without sustaining any injury. Although she maintained that her health had always been perfect, her husband reported that she had been admitted to a psychiatric hospital twice before they were married but he did not know any details of her treatment.

On examination she was over-active, disinhibited and paced repeatedly up and down the interview room. No abnormal signs were found in the cardiovascular system, chest or abdomen and there were no localising neurological signs. However the physical examination was conducted with great difficulty. She looked elated and described her mood as being very happy. She exhibited pressure of speech and flight of ideas, and believed herself to be a princess who had given birth to a future monarch. It was difficult to test her cognitive state because she was easily distracted by extraneous stimuli. She appeared perplexed but was correctly orientated in time and place. She performed poorly on the serial sevens test and the digit span test, being unable to repeat more than three digits forwards. She would not cooperate with other tests of cognition.

Screening test results

Haemoglobin	13.5 g/dl	ESR	8 mm/1st hr
WBC	5.9×10^9/l	MCV	90 fl
Potassium	4.0 mm/l	Sodium	140 mmol/l
Bicarbonate	25 mm/l	Chloride	97 mmol/l
Urea	4.7 mm/l	Creatinine	76 μmol/l
Calcium	2.20 mm/l	Phosphate	0.98 mmol/l
Total Protein	63 g/l	Albumin	35 g/l
Bilirubin	8 μmol/l		
Aspartate		Alkaline	
Transaminase	30 U/l	Phosphatase	73 U/l

Urine analysis: trace of protein

The Viva: questions and answers on page 132.

A student with jaundice

A 20-year-old English student presented with a 10-day history of yellowness of the skin. He had been perfectly well until two weeks previously, when he had experienced flu-like symptoms with malaise, generalised aching and nausea. He felt dreadful. He had a mild ache in the right upper part of his abdomen. He was a non-smoker. After four days, he had noticed his urine was dark and his stools pale, and next day his eyes were yellow. The yellowness had increased but his appetite had improved. There was slight itchiness of the skin. He had lost 4 kg weight during this illness.

Two months ago, he had been in Spain with his girl-friend on a camping holiday. He had eaten shellfish. His girl-friend was well and he knew of no other cases of jaundice. He denied drug abuse and had had no recent immunisations. He had had no recent dental treatment. He drank modest amounts of beer. He was living at home with his mother, father, younger brother and sister who were all well.

On examination, the patient appeared well and alert, but was deeply jaundiced. The liver edge could be felt 3 cm below the right costal margin on deep inspiration, and was tender. The spleen tip was palpable. There was no flapping tremor, vascular spiders, lymphadenopathy, oedema or ascites. He was not tattooed. Physical examination was otherwise normal.

Screening test results

Haemoglobin	14.3 g/dl	ESR	9 mm/1st hr
WBC	3.0×10^9/l	MCV	85 fl
Potassium	4.2 mmol/l	Sodium	136 mmol/l
Bicarbonate	26 mmol/l	Chloride	95 mmol/l
Urea	3.0 mmol/l	Creatinine	68 μmol/l
Calcium	2.42 mmol/l	Phosphate	1.15 mmol/l
Total Protein	78 g/l	Albumin	40 g/l
Bilirubin	119 μmol/l		
Aspartate		Alkaline	
Transaminase	620 U/l	Phosphatase	142 U/l

Urine analysis: bilirubin + + + ; urobilinogen −

The Viva: questions and answers on page 172.

Two years of diarrhoea

A 33-year-old single unemployed woman from Mauritius presented with a two-year history of diarrhoea. She reported that she opened her bowels three to four times each day, but the stool contained neither blood nor mucus. She thought that she passed a large volume of stool but she had not recognised any fat. For many years she had noticed intermittent mild mid-abdominal pain. She had lost weight, dropping from 60 to 50 kg in the preceding two years. She did not have nocturnal diarrhoea.

The patient had been diabetic for 10 years, treated with chlorpropamide.

On examination, the patient appeared thin and unwell. She was not ketotic. There was no abnormality in the cardiovascular or respiratory systems — in particular there was no evidence of diabetes-associated retinopathy, arterial or nervous system disease. Abdominal examination was unremarkable, except for marked vulvovaginitis due to candidiasis. Sigmoidoscopy revealed a healthy rectal mucosa, but the stool appeared greasy.

Screening test results

Haemoglobin	14.6 g/dl	ESR	9 mm/1st hr
WBC	6.7×10^9/l	MCV	85 fl
Potassium	4.4 mmol/l	Sodium	136 mmol/l
Bicarbonate	24 mmol/l	Chloride	95 mmol/l
Urea	3.7 mmol/l	Creatinine	69 μmol/l
Calcium	2.37 mmol/l	Phosphate	1.12 mmol/l
Total Protein	78 g/l	Albumin	45 g/l
Bilirubin	8 μmol/l		
Aspartate		Alkaline	
Transaminase	27 U/l	Phosphatase	48 U/l

Urine analysis: glucose + + +

The Viva: questions and answers on page 69.

'Pains in all my joints'

A 62-year-old male teacher presented with a six-month history of joint pains involving the small joints of his hands and feet, his wrists, shoulders, and both knees. His joints became extremely stiff and painful during the night, and he complained of troublesome tingling pain in both hands. It took until lunchtime each day before his joint stiffness diminished. During the previous six months he had lost 6 kg in weight, and had developed a dry cough with breathlessness on slight exertion. He had taken a variety of non-steroidal anti-inflammatory agents from his family doctor with little benefit.

On examination he had widespread polyarthritis, with swelling and tenderness of proximal interphalangeal and metacarpophalangeal joints, and synovitis of the dorsal tendon sheath. Both wrists were swollen and tender, with limitation of movement. His knees were swollen. All metatarsal heads were tender on compression. Neurological examination showed small muscle wasting in both hands and abduction of his right thumb was weak. There were no subcutaneous nodules. There was diminished movement of the chest, with dullness to percussion and absent breath sounds at the right base.

Screening test results

Haemoglobin	10.5 g/dl	ESR	110 mm/1st hr
WBC	11.5 × 10^9/l	MCV	80 fl
Potassium	3.6 mmol/l	Sodium	138 mmol/l
Bicarbonate	20 mmol/l	Chloride	110 mmol/l
Urea	6.2 mmol/l	Creatinine	86 μmol/l
Calcium	2.42 mmol/l	Phosphate	1.16 mmol/l
Total Protein	82 g/l	Albumin	38 g/l
Bilirubin	10 μmol/l		
Aspartate Transaminase	30 U/l	Alkaline Phosphatase	130 U/l

Urine analysis: normal

The Viva: questions and answers on page 148.

Septic feet

A 58-year-old female shop assistant presented with a four-day history of progressive drowsiness and confusion. A detailed history was not available from the patient, but her son revealed that she had been a diabetic on insulin for 30 years. Her diabetes had always been labile. Recent deterioration started a week prior to her presentation, when her toes became infected and began to discharge pus. Antibiotics prescribed by the family doctor did not help. Four days later she became anorexic, nauseated and began to vomit.

On examination, the patient was drowsy but responded to command. She was afebrile. Her hands and feet were cold, the skin inelastic and her tongue dry. The respiratory rate was 30/min. Her pulse rate was 112/min and the blood pressure was 95/55. Her foot pulses were absent on both sides; a purulent discharge was seen from the base of the right large and second toes. Ankle jerks were absent on both sides, and pressure on the Achilles tendon did not cause pain. Examination of the eyes, although difficult to perform, showed exudates, haemorrhages and two areas of new blood vessel formation.

Screening test results

Haemoglobin	16.2 g/dl	ESR	37 mm/1st hr
WBC	18.7 × 10⁹/l	MCV	8.3 fl
Potassium	3.2 mmol/l	Sodium	130 mmol/l
Bicarbonate	8 mmol/l	Chloride	85 mmol/l
Urea	18.3 mmol/l	Creatinine	248 μmol/l
Calcium	2.42 mmol/l	Phosphate	1.52 mmol/l
Total Protein	82 g/l	Albumin	33 g/l
Bilirubin	12 μmol/l		
Aspartate		Alkaline	
Transaminase	25 U/l	Phosphatase	87 U/l

Urine analysis: protein + + ; glucose + + + ; ketones + + +

The Viva: questions and answers on page 230.

Post-operative confusion

A 67-year-old retired train driver was admitted to a surgical ward for an elective cholecystectomy. For the past eight months he had been getting attacks of severe right-sided upper abdominal pain. He had a past history of chronic bronchitis and had one previous admission to hospital two years earlier with mild congestive cardiac failure. His current medication was frusemide 40 mg and digoxin 0.125 mg daily. His pre-operative haematology and biochemistry screens were normal.

Two days after admission to hospital he underwent an uneventful cholecystectomy. The common bile duct was clearly demonstrated and not dilated. A thickened and inflamed gall bladder containing several large stones was removed. Post-operatively he was given three litres of intravenous dextrose-saline daily.

Three days after his admission he became confused and on the fourth day he had a generalised convulsion.

On examination he was rousable but unable to talk rationally. He was able to obey simple commands. He was apyrexial and not cyanosed. The JVP was raised 2 cm. There was slight sacral oedema. The blood pressure was 130/70, both lying and standing. The pulse rate was 60/min and regular. Tissue perfusion was reasonably well maintained with the peripheries warm to palpation. Bilateral scattered basal crepitations were audible with occasional expiratory rhonchi. Abdominal examination revealed a healthy-looking abdominal wound. There was no abdominal distension. Scanty bowel sounds of normal quality were heard. Urine output had been maintained at between 750 and 1500 ml/24 hours.

Screening test results

Haemoglobin	11.2 g/dl	ESR	25 mm/1st hr
WBC	8.3×10^9/l	MCV	87 fl
Potassium	3.1 mmol/l	Sodium	109 mmol/l
Bicarbonate	12 mmol/l	Chloride	82 mmol/l
Urea	2.1 mmol/l	Creatinine	60 μmol/l
Calcium	2.04 mmol/l	Phosphate	0.82 mmol/l
Total Protein	65 g/l	Albumin	30 g/l
Bilirubin	17 μmol/l		
Aspartate		Alkaline	
Transaminase	55 U/l	Phosphatase	195 U/l

Urine analysis: normal

The Viva: questions and answers on page 87.

A sick sailor

A 30-year-old sailor from Trinidad became ill at sea with fever and headache. He had apparently enjoyed good health until this voyage, but there was a strong family history of tuberculosis. As soon as his ship docked, he was rushed to an infectious diseases hospital.

On examination, he had a temperature of 38.2°C and marked meningism. There was bilateral parotid enlargement and hepatosplenomegaly. Irido-cyclitis of the right eye prevented observation of the right optic disc, but there was papilloedoma in the left eye. There was slight right-sided facial weakness. The remainder of the clinical examination revealed no other abnormalities.

Screening test results

Haemoglobin	13.0 g/dl	ESR	73 mm/1st hr
WBC	10.1 × 10^9/l	MCV	84 fl
Potassium	3.9 mmol/l	Sodium	139 mmol/l
Bicarbonate	26 mmol/l	Chloride	101 mmol/l
Urea	6.1 mmol/l	Creatinine	79 μmol/l
Calcium	2.69 mmol/l	Phosphate	1.03 mmol/l
Total Protein	90 g/l	Albumin	37 g/l
Bilirubin	8 μmol/l		
Aspartate Transaminase	60 U/l	Alkaline Phosphatase	149 U/l

Urine analysis: normal

The Viva: questions and answers on page 181.

Pins and needles

A school teacher aged 25 noticed pins and needles in both feet with a feeling of constriction around her knees. The symptoms had been present for six weeks and had developed gradually. Symptoms were worse after walking and her right leg tended to become tired and to drag after half a mile. There was slight urgency of micturition. When taking a hot bath she noticed that temperature could not be felt in the left leg. Flexion of the neck produced a shower of pins and needles down the back and into both legs. She had experienced an episode of vertigo two years before, ascribed to vestibular neuronitis.

On examination there were no abnormal findings in the cranial nerves or arms. The legs showed slight weakness of hip flexion and of dorsiflexion of the right foot. Tone was increased slightly in both legs: all tendon reflexes were brisk, the right more than the left. Both plantar responses were extensor. Sensory testing showed diminished pinprick and thermal sensation over the left leg, extending to the trunk as high as the waist. There was reduced vibration and joint position sense in both legs. Back movements were full and painless; there was no spinal tenderness.

Screening test results

Haemoglobin	12.1 g/dl	ESR	9 mm/1st hr
WBC	$6.3 \times 10^9/l$	MCV	86 fl
Potassium	4.0 mmol/l	Sodium	139 mmol/l
Bicarbonate	28 mmol/l	Chloride	103 mmol/l
Urea	4.4 mmol/l	Creatinine	66 μmol/l
Calcium	2.31 mmol/l	Phosphate	1.13 mmol/l
Total Protein	70 g/l	Albumin	40 g/l
Bilirubin	9 μmol/l		
Aspartate		Alkaline	
Transaminase	17 U/l	Phosphatase	40 U/l

Urine analysis: normal

The Viva: questions and answers on page 142.

A confused patient

A 55-year-old club manager was admitted as an emergency in a confused state. Symptoms of headache, nausea and vomiting had developed during the two days before admission. Further history became available after initial treatment. In the preceding six months, he had noticed his skin was very sensitive, with extreme irritation when hot. A frontal headache had also been rather common during this time, which he put down to the pressure of work. He had some rather prolonged nose bleeds; however he had not noticed bleeding from any other site and he did not bruise easily. His appetite had been slightly reduced and he felt bloated after a meal. He smoked 20–30 cigarettes a day, but drank little alcohol. He took no drugs.

On examination the patient was confused, disorientated and very vague. Examination was difficult as he withdrew when he was touched. He was markedly plethoric with prominent capillaries on his nose and cheeks, the mucous membranes were deeply red. His lips were cyanosed. There was no clubbing. His blood pressure was 165/90. Both the liver and spleen extended below the costal margin, by 2 cm and 5 cm respectively. Neurological examination suggested meningeal irritation, but no focal lesion could be demonstrated. Retinal examination showed distended veins but no haemorrhages.

Screening test results

Haemoglobin	22.4 g/dl	ESR	1 mm/1st hr
WBC	$20.3 \times 10^9/l$	MCV	73 fl
Potassium	3.7 mmol/l	Sodium	140 mmol/l
Bicarbonate	30 mmol/l	Chloride	97 mmol/l
Urea	5.5 mmol/l	Creatinine	89 μmol/l
Calcium	2.32 mmol/l	Phosphate	1.09 mmol/l
Total Protein	67 g/l	Albumin	36 g/l
Bilirubin	12 μmol/l		
Aspartate		Alkaline	
Transaminase	37 U/l	Phosphatase	61 U/l

Urine analysis: normal

The Viva: questions and answers on page 162.

Sudden breathlessness

A 65-year-old senior executive reported that, when on holiday three weeks previously, he was climbing a cliff path and experienced a sudden onset of breathlessness. This was severe and, although he immediately sat down and rested, it lasted for about 15 minutes. Until this episode he had been asymptomatic, but it appeared that he had been voluntarily limiting his activities for some months. He was unaware that the strength of his heart had previously been questioned; however he had been rejected for military service at the start of World War Two. There was no history of rheumatic fever.

On examination, he was a well-preserved, elderly man. He was in sinus rhythm. The carotid pulse was slow rising, with an early notch and a thrill of the upstroke. There was a 3 cm 'a' wave on the venous pulse. The apex beat was sustained, with a double impulse. On auscultation, there was an ejection systolic murmur down the left sternal edge, and what appeared to be a separate ejection systolic murmur at the apex. The second sound was single and audible at the apex, as well as at the base of the heart. The peripheral pulses were all present and equal. Other systems were normal.

Screening test results

Haemoglobin	15.0 g/dl	ESR	5 mm/1st hr
WBC	7.5×10^9/l	MCV	90 fl
Potassium	4.2 mmol/l	Sodium	137 mmol/l
Bicarbonate	25 mmol/l	Chloride	104 mmol/l
Urea	3.5 mmol/l	Creatinine	78 μmol/l
Calcium	2.40 mmol/l	Phosphate	1.00 mmol/l
Total Protein	75 g/l	Albumin	45 g/l
Bilirubin	14 μmol/l		
Aspartate		Alkaline	
Transaminase	22 U/l	Phosphatase	52 U/l

Urine analysis: normal

The Viva: questions and answers on page 115.

A mite too small

A 12-year-old boy was keen on rugby and horse-riding. However, he was smaller than the rest of his class and he became short of breath whenever he exercised. His parents were worried about him as he had been troubled from infancy with recurrent coughs and colds, which always turned into bronchitis with wheezing. He often coughed during the night. He had been to the family doctor, but had never been admitted to hospital.

On examination he was thin and obviously small for his age. His chest was hyperinflated and the lower ribs and costal margins were splayed out. He also had excoriated eczema at the flexures of the elbows and wrists.

Screening test results

Haemoglobin	12.1 g/dl	ESR	4 mm/1st hr
WBC	6.9×10^9/l	MCV	94 fl
Potassium	3.7 mmol/l	Sodium	139 mmol/l
Bicarbonate	27 mmol/l	Chloride	99 mmol/l
Urea	4.2 mmol/l	Creatinine	61 μmol/l
Calcium	2.50 mmol/l	Phosphate	1.01 mmol/l
Total Protein	67 g/l	Albumin	43 g/l
Bilirubin	9 μmol/l		
Aspartate		Alkaline	
Transaminase	21 U/l	Phosphatase	147 U/l

Urine analysis: normal

The Viva: questions and answers on page 220.

Palpitations and dizziness

A 37-year-old married woman presented with a 12-month history of acute, recurrent episodes of palpitations, dizziness, and breathlessness associated with a tight constricting feeling around her chest. Each episode lasted between five and ten minutes and was accompanied by feelings of intense anxiety so that the patient thought she was going to die from a heart attack. Initially they had occurred every two or three weeks but they had become progressively more frequent and, at the time of her presentation, they were occurring nearly every day. She had had to give up her part-time secretarial job and was unable to cope with some of her domestic responsibilities, including meeting her children from school and doing the family shopping in a local supermarket unless her husband accompanied her.

On physical examination she had a sinus tachycardia, 100/min and her blood pressure was 140/95; her blood pressure fell to 130/80 by the end of the interview. Otherwise physical examination was completely normal.

Screening test results

Haemoglobin	13.4 g/dl	ESR	5 mm/1st hr
WBC	$5.9 \times 10^9/l$	MCV	101 fl
Potassium	4.1 mmol/l	Sodium	140 mmol/l
Bicarbonate	25 mmol/l	Chloride	99 mmol/l
Urea	3.6 mmol/l	Creatinine	79 μmol/l
Calcium	2.19 mmol/l	Phosphate	1.12 mmol/l
Total Protein	71 g/l	Albumin	44 g/l
Bilirubin	11 μmol/l		
Aspartate		Alkaline	
Transaminase	32 U/l	Phosphatase	75 U/l

Urine analysis: normal

The Viva: questions and answers on page 203.

Progressive jaundice

A 76-year-old retired lorry driver had previously enjoyed good health. However, he presented to his general practitioner with a three-week history of polydipsia and polyuria. Glycosuria was detected. The fasting blood glucose concentration was raised and was still increased two hours after an oral glucose load. There was no family history of diabetes mellitus. He had never had his urine tested previously for glucose. At that time he was said to have an enlarged liver. He had lost 5 kg in weight. His diabetes mellitus was treated with carbohydrate restriction and insulin.

Two months later he was referred to hospital because of the slow onset of jaundice, which had progressed and deepened over the previous four weeks. The stools had become pale and the urine had darkened. He was troubled by itching of the skin, which was only partially relieved by antihistamines. There was no abdominal pain. He was apyrexial. He took no drugs apart from insulin. He had lost 10 kg in weight over the past six months.

Examination revealed an elderly, frail, and jaundiced man. He weighed 50 kg. He had clearly lost much flesh recently. Scratch marks were obvious on the skin. Examination of the abdomen showed a smooth, non-tender liver edge 10 cm below the right costal margin. There was a possible oval, non-tender mass projecting from the liver edge; this might have been the gall-bladder. The spleen was not palpable and there was no ascites.

Screening test results

Haemoglobin	11.7 g/dl	ESR	40 mm/1st hr
WBC	9.6 × 10⁹/l	MCV	74 fl
Potassium	2.7 mmol/l	Sodium	138 mmol/l
Bicarbonate	24 mmol/l	Chloride	95 mmol/l
Urea	2.9 mmol/l	Creatinine	78 μmol/l
Calcium	2.50 mmol/l	Phosphate	1.15 mmol/l
Total Protein	63 g/l	Albumin	34 g/l
Bilirubin	296 μmol/l		
Aspartate Transaminase	347 U/l	Alkaline Phosphatase	2055 U/l

Urine analysis: bilirubin + + + ; urobilinogen − ; glucose −

The Viva: questions and answers on page 92.

A psychiatric problem

A 28-year-old woman complained of increasing obesity. Two years earlier she had been admitted to a mental hospital with schizophrenia. She was treated with depot injections of a phenothiazine (fluphenazine) and gained 15 kg in weight. She had noticed difficulty in climbing the stairs, and complained that her menstrual periods had ceased.

On examination the patient was obese, and mildly hypertensive (blood pressure 155/100). She had a soft skin with striae over her abdomen, buttocks and breasts. She had excessive hair over her face. There was weakness of the limb-girdle muscles, but the reflexes were intact.

Screening test results

Haemoglobin	15.5 g/dl	ESR	5 mm/1st hr
WBC	9.7 × 10⁹/l	MCV	82 fl
Potassium	3.0 mmol/l	Sodium	145 mmol/l
Bicarbonate	31 mmol/l	Chloride	102 mmol/l
Urea	4.9 mmol/l	Creatinine	71 μmol/l
Calcium	2.29 mmol/l	Phosphate	1.08 mmol/l
Total Protein	72 g/l	Albumin	38 g/l
Bilirubin	7 μmol/l		
Aspartate		Alkaline	
Transaminase	23 U/l	Phosphatase	75 U/l

Urine analysis: glucose +

The Viva: questions and answers on page 187.

Early exhaustion

For four months, a 46-year-old male lorry driver had noticed increasing weakness, palpitations, and early exhaustion. He reported retrosternal discomfort on exertion. He also complained of anorexia; over the past two months he had lost 12 kg weight. For the last month he observed that he was yellow. Direct questioning brought out the fact that his tongue had been sore for a year and that he had recently experienced retrosternal chest pain when walking. His urine was very dark but the bowel motions were a normal colour. Normally he consumed four to five pints of beer a day, but he had lost the taste for this as he felt bloated after a beer. He was not taking any drugs, had never been transfused and had never been abroad. He ate a normal diet.

On examination, he was extremely pale and mildly jaundiced; he had clearly lost weight. His pulse rate was 120/min, the JVP was raised 1 cm, and he had an ejection systolic murmur. There was no ankle or sacral oedema. His tongue was smooth. The spleen could be felt 4 cm below the costal margin. No abnormal neurological signs were found.

Screening test results

Haemoglobin	4.2 g/dl	ESR	27 mm/1st hr
WBC	4.1 × 10⁹/l	MCV	118 fl
Potassium	4.6 mmol/l	Sodium	136 mmol/l
Bicarbonate	23 mmol/l	Chloride	99 mmol/l
Urea	4.6 mmol/l	Creatinine	78 μmol/l
Calcium	2.43 mmol/l	Phosphate	1.25 mmol/l
Total Protein	76 g/l	Albumin	43 g/l
Bilirubin	44 μmol/l		
Aspartate		Alkaline	
Transaminase	7 U/l	Phosphatase	47 U/l

Urine analysis: urobilinogen + + +

The Viva: questions and answers on page 75.

Loss of weight and height

A 55-year-old heavy-smoking taxi driver developed recurrent respiratory tract infections throughout one winter and they continued to recur during the following summer, despite a sunny Mediterranean holiday. He also suffered two separate episodes of urinary tract infection. In the course of one year he had lost height, for he no longer hit his head when entering his small kitchen. During the last three months he had developed low-backache and prostatic symptoms. One month ago he developed *Herpes zoster* on the trunk.

On examination he appeared older than his age, possibly because he was just recovering from an attack of purulent bronchitis. There were scattered added sounds in both lung fields. There was an area of healing *Herpes zoster* over the left loin. There was moderate enlargement of the prostate. Sigmoidoscopy was normal.

Screening test results

Haemoglobin	7.9 g/dl	ESR	80 mm/1st hr
WBC	12.2 × 10^9/l	MCV	86 fl
Potassium	3.8 mmol/l	Sodium	127 mmol/l
Bicarbonate	26 mmol/l	Chloride	95 mmol/l
Urea	9.8 mmol/l	Creatinine	142 μmol/l
Calcium	2.92 mmol/l	Phosphate	0.79 mmol/l
Total Protein	95 g/l	Albumin	35 g/l
Bilirubin	8 μmol/l		
Aspartate		Alkaline	
Transaminase	21 U/l	Phosphatase	32 U/l

Urine analysis: albumin +

The Viva: questions and answers on page 125.

Double vision

An 18-year-old female clerk presented to an eye department complaining of double vision for six weeks. The images were separated vertically and worse on looking upwards to the right. On direct questioning she admitted to tiredness on chewing, and pain in the neck with a tendency for the head to fall forwards. There were no symptoms in the limbs and no relevant past history. She had general lassitude with weight loss of 2 kg. There was no bowel disturbance.

On examination, she was anxious but afebrile with a pulse rate of 80 in sinus rhythm. She had a fine finger tremor but no thyroid enlargement. In the nervous system there was slight ptosis on the left side; she had vertical diplopia on looking upwards to the right, the false image was from the right eye. There was no proptosis, lid retraction or lid lag. There was weakness of the obicularis oculi muscles on both sides. She could not forcibly extend the head against resistance. The limbs were normal except for some weakness of abduction in both shoulders. The reflexes were preserved and sensation was intact.

Screening test results

Haemoglobin	13.0 g/dl	ESR	2 mm/1st hr
WBC	6.3 × 10⁹/l	MCV	92 fl
Potassium	3.8 mmol/l	Sodium	138 mmol/l
Bicarbonate	29 mmol/l	Chloride	100 mmol/l
Urea	6.3 mmol/l	Creatinine	98 μmol/l
Calcium	2.49 mmol/l	Phosphate	1.01 mmol/l
Total Protein	77 g/l	Albumin	47 g/l
Bilirubin	12 μmol/l		
Aspartate		Alkaline	
Transaminase	32 U/l	Phosphatase	74 U/l

Urine analysis: normal

The Viva: questions and answers on page 63.

Holiday stomach upset

A 27-year-old unmarried secretary went on holiday to North Africa with a group of young people. Everybody developed diarrhoea and vomiting at some stage of the holiday, but all recovered promptly except the patient. She complained that for the next month she continued to feel ill, with an uncomfortable distended stomach and continuing diarrhoea. She opened her bowels five times a day, especially after meals, but noticed neither blood nor mucus. She was already thin and her weight dropped from 53 to 47 kg.

She gave no history of any serious illness. Since she started menstruating she had had repeated courses of iron tablets for anaemia. Her periods were not heavy, and she had never taken the contraceptive pill. The family doctor's letter said that her haemoglobin had ranged from 8.2 to 11.2 g/dl. She had one course of iron injections, but had received only iron tablets for the preceding year.

On examination the patient appeared thin but healthy. There was no significant abnormality in the cardiovascular or respiratory systems, apart from a quiet systolic ejection murmur. The abdomen was slightly distended, without any palpable masses or organs. The anus appeared healthy; the rectal mucosa was normal at sigmoidoscopy.

Screening test results

Haemoglobin	9.8 g/dl	ESR	12 mm/1st hr
WBC	4.7×10^9/l	MCV	104 fl
Potassium	3.9 mmol/l	Sodium	136 mmol/l
Bicarbonate	29 mmol/l	Chloride	98 mmol/l
Urea	3.7 mmol/l	Creatinine	82 μmol/l
Calcium	2.12 mmol/l	Phosphate	0.70 mmol/l
Total Protein	67 g/l	Albumin	32 g/l
Bilirubin	12 μmol/l		
Aspartate		Alkaline	
Transaminase	35 U/l	Phosphatase	147 U/l

Urine analysis: normal

The Viva: questions and answers on page 206.

Loin pain and fever

A 19-year-old nurse presented with a history of malaise for three days, with left loin pain for the preceding 24 hours. On the day that she presented she noticed a high fever, which was followed by a rigor. She had nocturnal enuresis until the age of 14. She gave a long history of urgency of micturition, and had been occasionally incontinent of urine for as long as she could remember. Her last menstrual period was 15 weeks earlier: she was probably pregnant.

On examination she looked unwell. Her temperature was 39.5°C. She was restless and a little confused. Blood pressure 90/60, pulse 140 and regular. She was flushed with warm, well-perfused peripheries. Abdominal examination revealed tenderness and guarding in the left loin. There was fullness in the left flank and spasm of the left lumbar paraspinal muscles. There was a firm palpable mass arising out of the pelvis which extended to midway between the umbilicus and the pubic symphysis.

A neurological examination, performed after she had recovered from her acute illness, was abnormal. Her ankle jerks were absent and there was diminished sensation for light touch over the lateral border of both feet. Vibration sense was lacking below the middle of both tibia. The rest of her neurological examination was essentially normal.

Screening test results

Haemoglobin	10.8 g/dl	ESR	43 mm/1st hr
WBC	$17.4 \times 10^9/l$	MCV	86 fl
Potassium	4.5 mmol/l	Sodium	140 mmol/l
Bicarbonate	22 mmol/l	Chloride	98 mmol/l
Urea	14.2 mmol/l	Creatinine	180 μmol/l
Calcium	2.41 mmol/l	Phosphate	0.9 mmol/l
Total Protein	67 g/l	Albumin	39 g/l
Bilirubin	5 μmol/l		
Aspartate		Alkaline	
Transaminase	12 U/l	Phosphatase	73 U/l

Urine analysis: blood trace; protein + +

The Viva: questions and answers on page 151.

Epileptic fit

A 38-year-old male organist became progressively ill over six months. He lost weight, developed an irritating cough, and gradually became confused. He only presented to a doctor when he had an epileptic fit, whilst playing the organ during morning service.

On admission to hospital he had already regained consciousness, but he remained drowsy and confused. He had nicotine-stained fingers, but no clubbing. His pulse was 96 in sinus rhythm, with a blood pressure of 160/105 both lying and standing. There were absent breath sounds over the right lung. The remainder of the physical examination was normal; in particular there was no neurological abnormality.

Screening test results

Haemoglobin	10.1 g/dl	ESR	49 mm/1st hr
WBC	10.2×10^9/l	MCV	83 fl
Potassium	3.0 mmol/l	Sodium	112 mmol/l
Bicarbonate	26 mmol/l	Chloride	84 mmol/l
Urea	2.9 mmol/l	Creatinine	54 μmol/l
Calcium	2.47 mmol/l	Phosphate	0.87 mmol/l
Total Protein	67 g/l	Albumin	38 g/l
Bilirubin	8 μmol/l		
Aspartate Transaminase	39 U/l	Alkaline Phosphatase	83 U/l

Urine analysis: normal

The Viva: questions and answers on page 112.

Impaired speech and memory

A 60-year-old right-handed hospital administrator noticed the loss of verbal fluency and a difficulty in recalling names of common objects. Colleagues remarked on the failure of his memory and a decline in his previously high standards of work. The condition progressed over three months. There was a past history of classical migraine and bilateral acute otitis media in childhood. He had occasional discharge from the left ear and was deaf on that side.

On examination he appeared alert and intelligent. He made a number of mistakes in naming common objects and tended to transpose syllables when writing. His immediate recall of a sequence of numbers was normal, but he was unable to remember a name and address after five minutes. The optic discs were normal but there was no venous pulsation. On confrontation there was restriction in the upper temporal visual field in the right eye and the upper nasal field in the left eye. He had a mild right lower facial weakness and a conduction-type deafness in the left ear. The limbs showed no weakness. There was a slight increase of reflexes in the right arm and leg. The right plantar response was extensor. There was a chronic perforation of the left ear drum.

Screening test results

Haemoglobin	13.0 g/dl	ESR	7 mm/1st hr
WBC	6.7 × 10^9/l	MCV	94 fl
Potassium	4.2 mmol/l	Sodium	139 mmol/l
Bicarbonate	27 mmol/l	Chloride	99 mmol/l
Urea	6.0 mmol/l	Creatinine	107 μmol/l
Calcium	2.50 mmol/l	Phosphate	1.01 mmol/l
Total Protein	76 g/l	Albumin	45 g/l
Bilirubin	12 μmol/l		
Aspartate		Alkaline	
Transaminase	27 U/l	Phosphatase	103 U/l

Urine analysis: normal

The Viva: questions and answers on page 233.

Pyrexia and breathlessness

A 30-year-old disc jockey was admitted with a six-week history of malaise, initially diagnosed as influenza. He was given a short course of ampicillin with some improvement. However, his symptoms recurred and were accompanied by night sweats. At the time of admission, he also complained of mild breathlessness on exertion. Over the succeeding five days, his breathlessness became progressively more severe, and was accompanied by orthopnoea and paroxysmal nocturnal dyspnoea. It failed to respond to digitalisation and increasing doses of oral, and finally of intravenous, frusemide.

On examination, he looked ill and was breathless at rest. He had a temperature of 39.4°C. There was neither clubbing of the fingers nor any splinter haemorrhage. He was in sinus rhythm, with a blood pressure of 110/40. The pulse volume was increased, but its character was normal. Du Rosiez' sign was positive (a diastolic murmur was audible over the femoral artery, when it was partially compressed by the thumb). The venous pressure was increased to 4 cm, with a dominant 'v' wave. The praecordial impulse was very active, although the apex was not sustained. On auscultation, a soft systolic murmur was audible in the aortic area. There were no diastolic murmurs, although a low-pitched early diastolic sound, similar to a third heart sound, was audible at the apex. There were crepitations at the lung bases, but no peripheral oedema. Abdominal palpation was difficult, but the spleen was probably enlarged 2 cm below the costal margin. The peripheral pulses were present and equal, and the optic fundi were normal.

Screening test results

Haemoglobin	8.5 g/dl	ESR	96 mm/1st hr
WBC	25 × 10⁹/l	MCV	75 fl
Potassium	3.3 mmol/l	Sodium	120 mmol/l
Bicarbonate	18 mmol/l	Chloride	85 mmol/l
Urea	10.5 mmol/l	Creatinine	140 μmol/l
Calcium	2.00 mmol/l	Phosphate	1.2 mmol/l
Total Protein	55 g/l	Albumin	35 g/l
Bilirubin	20 μmol/l		
Aspartate		Alkaline	
Transaminase	35 U/l	Phosphatase	80 U/l

Urine analysis: protein +; blood + +

The Viva: questions and answers on page 103.

Nausea and vomiting

A 68-year-old retired school mistress became progressively nauseated and anorexic. She started to vomit after meals, and was losing weight. She had no history of indigestion or abdominal pain, no headache, and she denied any other symptoms. She had always enjoyed good health and this was the first time that she had seen a doctor for many years.

On examination, the patient was unwell and slightly dehydrated. The remainder of the physical examination was completely normal.

Screening test results

Haemoglobin	16.6 g/dl	ESR	13 mm/1st hr
WBC	4.7 × 10^9/l	MCV	94 fl
Potassium	3.8 mmol/l	Sodium	135 mmol/l
Bicarbonate	27 mmol/l	Chloride	111 mmol/l
Urea	10.1 mmol/l	Creatinine	127 μmol/l
Calcium	3.82 mmol/l	Phosphate	0.62 mmol/l
Total Protein	78 g/l	Albumin	44 g/l
Bilirubin	14 μmol/l		
Aspartate		Alkaline	
Transaminase	32 U/l	Phosphatase	120 U/l

Urine analysis: normal

The Viva: questions and answers on page 120.

Prolonged ill health

A 45-year-old man had a vague history of malaise. He found it increasingly hard to cope with his work as an accountant, and his wife noticed that he fell asleep most evenings. For the last three months he had been eating poorly and had lost about 5 kg in weight. For a month he noticed difficulty when getting out of a chair, and to climb the stairs at night he had to pull himself up by the banisters. He had been sleeping poorly and was scratching at night. A life insurance examination 15 years earlier revealed mild hypertension but no medical follow-up had been arranged.

On examination he was pale and sallow. His skin was dry and there were numerous scratch marks over his elbows and legs. The blood pressure was 190/115. There was no evidence of fluid overload. Examination of the fundi showed only arteriovenous nipping. The chest and abdomen were unremarkable. Neurological examination revealed a marked weakness of hip flexion: the patient was unable to sit up from the lying position without using his arms. Vibration sense was absent from both feet, and the ankle jerks could not be elicited.

Screening test results

Haemoglobin	5.3 g/dl	ESR	31 mm/1st hr
WBC	4.6×10^9/l	MCV	89 fl
Potassium	6.1 mmol/l	Sodium	139 mmol/l
Bicarbonate	10 mmol/l	Chloride	90 mmol/l
Urea	55 mmol/l	Creatinine	1850 μmol/l
Calcium	1.40 mmol/l	Phosphate	2.31 mmol/l
Total Protein	65 g/l	Albumin	29 g/l
Bilirubin	7 μmol/l		
Aspartate		Alkaline	
Transaminase	21 U/l	Phosphatase	248 U/l

Urine analysis: protein + ; glucose 1 per cent

The Viva: questions and answers on page 226.

Anaemia on anticoagulants

A 75-year-old retired army officer had been attending the anticoagulant clinic regularly since 1961, when he was put on phenindione following a right ileo-femoral endarterectomy. During the next 17 years he experienced no further trouble with that leg.

However, his general practitioner referred him back to the clinic because the patient was becoming increasingly short of breath on exertion and he looked very pale. He did not complain of dyspepsia, loss of weight or change in bowel habit; any history of blood-streaked or melaena stools was denied. During his army life he had not suffered from any tropical diseases.

On examination, he was an impeccably-dressed fit-looking man, who was clinically anaemic. A number of large telangiectatic lesions were present on the buccal mucous membranes, on the underside of the tongue, on the soft palate, and on the palmar surface of his fingers. He was not in heart failure and his blood pressure was 180/95. His abdomen was soft, no masses were felt, the liver was not enlarged, but a dark stool was found on rectal examination (he was already on iron). Apart from absent ankle jerks, the neurological examination was normal.

Screening test results

Haemoglobin	9.3 g/dl	ESR	10 mm/1st hr
WBC	$10.9 \times 10^9/l$	MCV	69 fl
Potassium	4.3 mmol/l	Sodium	146 mmol/l
Bicarbonate	27 mmol/l	Chloride	102 mmol/l
Urea	4.4 mmol/l	Creatinine	108 μmol/l
Calcium	2.52 mmol/l	Phosphate	1.13 mmol/l
Total Protein	67 g/l	Albumin	39 g/l
Bilirubin	7 μmol/l		
Aspartate		Alkaline	
Transaminase	19 U/l	Phosphatase	49 U/l

Urine analysis: normal

The Viva: questions and answers on page 144.

Part 2: The Viva

Double vision

WHAT IS THE DIFFERENTIAL DIAGNOSIS?

1   Myasthenia gravis
    Ocular myopathy
    Myasthenic (Eaton-Lambert) syndrome

Myasthenia gravis may start at any age in either sex, but it is commonest in young women. Muscles of the head and neck are involved early, especially chewing, swallowing, phonation and extraocular muscles. Patchy involvement is characteristic of myasthenia gravis: in this case the superior rectus muscle of the right eye was involved, while other ocular muscles were spared.

Ocular myopathy usually produces a symmetrical weakness with severe limitation of eye movements, bilateral ptosis but usually no diplopia. It may be familial.

The myasthenic (Eaton-Lambert) syndrome is usually associated with carcinoma, but there are many exceptions. The limbs, rather than the face or eyes, are characteristically involved early. Tendon reflexes are depressed and the electromyogram shows typical post-tetanic potentiation.

Polymyositis seldom involves the ocular muscles but may cause facial and limb weakness. Often muscle pain and tenderness are present. Multiple sclerosis usually produces a gaze palsy rather than an individual muscle weakness. Bilateral facial weakness would also be most unusual. Partial 3rd nerve palsy could explain diplopia but not the other features. Although some forms of polyneuritis preferentially affect cranial nerves, they are usually associated with sensory changes and with signs in the limbs.

WHAT ADDITIONAL INVESTIGATIONS WOULD YOU CONSIDER?

1   Tensilon test (edrophonium test)
10 mg edrophonium given intravenously markedly improved this patient's power in the neck and abolished diplopia. This strongly suggests myasthenia gravis, although either the myasthenic syndrome or polymyositis may occasionally be improved a little by the anti-cholinesterase. Intravenous atropine should always be immediately available when using Tensilon.

2   Acetylcholine receptor antibody
The antibody was present in a titre greater than 1/100. This test is positive in about 90 per cent of patients with generalised myasthenia,

but it is less reliable in ocular myasthenia. Between patients the titre is unrelated to severity of disease although in an individual patient a rising titre suggests worsening disease. The titres of other organ-specific antibodies may be raised; a high titre of striated muscle antibody is found in patients with thymoma.

3 Chest X-ray and/or CT scan

No abnormality was seen in the thoracic cavity. Myasthenia gravis is sometimes associated with tumour or hyperplasia of the thymus which may be visible on a plain film or CT scan. Retrosternal thyroid enlargement may also be seen.

4 Plasma thyroxine

It is necessary to rule out hyperthyroidism coexisting with myasthenia gravis: this patient was euthyroid with a plasma thyroxine of 90 nmol/l (normal range 66–133 nmol/l).

5 Electromyogram (EMG)

In most patients with generalised myasthenia, a reduction in the size of muscle-action potential occurs with repetitive nerve stimulation (3/sec). In this case, no abnormality was found.

WHAT IS THE FINAL DIAGNOSIS?

Myasthenia gravis.

HOW WOULD YOU MANAGE THIS PATIENT?

Treatment should be started with pyridostigmine 60 mg tds, increasing to six times daily. This caused some improvement in this patient's symptoms, but she was still easily fatigued and unable to lead a normal life. Thymectomy was advised after six months of medical treatment; a hyperplastic thymus was removed. Post-operatively there was some reduction in the pyridostigmine dosage, but no marked improvement in the muscle power for the first six months. Subsequently slow and steady improvement has occurred.

COMMENT

Prednisolone (25 mg per day increasing to 100 mg per day on alternate days) will often improve muscle power, but it is unsatisfactory as a long-term treatment for young patients. Immunosuppressive treatment (azathioprine) is useful in patients who show incomplete response to thymectomy, but it may take many months before its full benefit is seen. Thymectomy is the most satisfactory treatment for myasthenia gravis: the majority of patients show a response although this may also be delayed for some months.

Good prognostic features are: being a female patient, being a young patient, and the discovery of a hyperplastic thymus at thymectomy.

Plasmapheresis causes dramatic, although temporary, improvement in muscle power. It is useful as a preparation for surgery in patients with respiratory muscle weakness.

EXAMINERS' FOLLOW-UP QUESTIONS

1 Why is myasthenia gravis now regarded as an autoimmune disease?
2 What special precautions are required when a myasthenic patient becomes pregnant?
3. What is a cholinergic crisis and how is it treated?
4 What special instructions should be given to the nurses when caring for a patient with severe myasthenia, weakness of speech and swallowing?
5 What late effects may follow the removal of the thymus gland in childhood?

R.W.R.R.

Tachypnoea

WHAT IS THE DIFFERENTIAL DIAGNOSIS?

1   Pulmonary embolism
    Pleurodynia
    Pleurisy due to infection
      Bronchopneumonia
      Lobar pneumonia
      Tuberculosis

Pleurisy can provide a major diagnostic problem — particularly for the family doctor who does not have the benefit of immediate investigations. The family doctor also had the disadvantage of not knowing that this girl was receiving the contraceptive pill from a clinic: only the 'anonymous' house physician elicited this fact.

  The screening tests reveal a low ESR and normal haemoglobin, which make tuberculosis unlikely, and a white cell count less than $15 \times 10^9/l$, which makes a pyogenic chest infection unlikely. However, it is difficult to get a more precise diagnosis without further investigations.

WHAT ADDITIONAL INVESTIGATIONS WOULD YOU CONSIDER?

1   Chest X-ray
The chest X-ray revealed an elevated right diaphragm (5 cm above the left), but the lung fields appeared clear. There was a small pleural effusion on the right.

2   ECG
The ECG showed acute right ventricular 'strain' with T wave inversion in leads V1–V4 and right bundle-branch block. The classical S1, Q3, T3 pattern was found in the standard limb leads. This combination of changes is classical of acute pulmonary embolism.

3   Arterial blood gases
The patient had low oxygen and carbon dioxide tension. These findings would be very unusual in an otherwise healthy girl, but are not specific for pulmonary infarction. They may also be found in any of the pulmonary infections, if sufficiently severe.

4   Ventilation-perfusion lung scans
Pulmonary scans use technetium-labelled microspheres to demonstrate the pulmonary circulation and inhaled krypton[81] to identify alveolar ventilation. The classical picture of pulmonary embolism

shows one or more defects in the pulmonary circulation, with completely normal ventilation of both lung fields. Thus, the pulmonary infarct shows as a ventilation-perfusion mismatch.

The lung scan should not be performed if the chest X-ray is already abnormal, for results are difficult to interpret if there is pre-existing lung disease. A normal perfusion scan and a normal chest X-ray eliminate the diagnosis of pulmonary embolism.

This patient did have an abnormal perfusion scan with two discrete defects in the right lung, with a normal ventilation scan.

5 Pulmonary arteriogram

This is a reliable but invasive technique that is only available in specialist centres. The investigation is particularly indicated if the patient is critically ill and the diagnosis is in doubt; or if pulmonary embolectomy is being considered; or if the patient has pre-existing pulmonary or cardiovascular disease. As this test is usually performed only in patients who are gravely ill, it is often possible to see large thrombi in major pulmonary vessels.

6. Leg venograms

Venograms of the legs can demonstrate the deep venous system up to the inferior vena cava. Unfortunately, the technique is painful and may even provoke further thrombosis. It should be reserved for those patients where the diagnosis is really in doubt.

WHAT IS THE FINAL DIAGNOSIS?

Pulmonary embolism, probably associated with an oral contraceptive.

HOW WOULD YOU MANAGE THIS PATIENT?

Although this patient has had pulmonary embolism, the circulation is not compromised and she has an adequate cardiac output.

The major objective of treatment is to stop the propagation of existing thrombosis, and further thrombo-embolism. The patient should be anticoagulated. Before any anticoagulant is given, the prothrombin time should be checked to make sure that there is no pre-existing abnormality of coagulation.

Heparin is best given by an infusion pump at a rate of 1000 U/hr, or much less satisfactorily as 10 000 U every six hours, or 5000 U every four hours. If heparin is infused for more than 48 hours, the patient's thrombin time should be checked. The thrombin time should be prolonged to between twice and seven times normal.

After five days of treatment with heparin, the patient should be anticoagulated using warfarin, which should be continued for three to six months.

An alternative strategy for a patient who has survived a massive pulmonary embolism is to use streptokinase or urokinase, which will speed the lysis of the emboli. Both drugs can produce catastrophic changes in blood clotting, and should only be used in specialised centres.

Pulmonary embolectomy should be reserved for those patients who have persisting hypotension due to obstruction of the pulmonary circulation.

Finally, this patient should be encouraged not only to stop smoking but also to abandon using the oral contraceptive.

COMMENT

The three factors thought to predispose to vascular thrombosis are reduction in blood flow, damage to the vessel wall, and increased coagulability of the blood. Contributing factors include bedrest or immobility; surgery, trauma or burns; previous venous thrombosis or cardiac disease; and obesity or paralytic disorders.

Uncommon non-thrombotic pulmonary embolism may be caused by air, fat, malignant cells, amniotic fluid, parasites or foreign material.

The physician must be aware that thrombo-embolism is probably very common in hospital patients. If there is no pulmonary infarction the only symptoms may be breathlessness, tachycardia, anxiety and restlessness. If there is pulmonary infarction the symptoms will be much as observed in this patient but, by the time the patient develops haemodynamic impairment, there is probably 30–50 per cent obstruction of the pulmonary vascular bed.

EXAMINERS' FOLLOW-UP QUESTIONS

1 To what type of embolism are jockeys prone?
2 What is the common type of pulmonary infarction in the West Indies?
3 What are the consequences of several repeated minor pulmonary emboli?
4 Describe the lungs of drug addicts.
5 What analgesic, hypnotic and H_2-antagonist would you recommend for a patient on warfarin?

D.G.J.

Two years of diarrhoea

WHAT IS THE DIFFERENTIAL DIAGNOSIS?

1 Diarrhoea (probably steatorrhoea)
    Pancreatic disease — chronic pancreatitis
    Giardiasis
    Coeliac disease
    Tropical sprue
    Bacterial overgrowth of small bowel
    Intestinal tuberculosis
2 Diabetes mellitus

The combination of profound steatorrhoea (that can be recognised on sigmoidoscopy), abdominal .pain and diabetes mellitus strongly suggests pancreatic disease. Chronic pancreatitis is more likely in a young patient than carcinoma of the pancreas.

Other causes of steatorrhoea should also be considered — the normal haemoglobin, ESR and albumin make them all much less likely than pancreatic disease.

Diarrhoea and malabsorption can be due to diabetic autonomic neuropathy with bacterial overgrowth in a relatively stagnant small intestine. This patient had no evidence of autonomic neuropathy — for example, postural hypotension.

WHAT ADDITIONAL INVESTIGATIONS WOULD YOU CONSIDER?

1 Three-day faecal fat
On a 70 g fat diet the patient's three-day sample weighed 1090 g and contained 96 mmol of fat/day (normal < 18.0). The weight of the stools confirmed the patient's history of diarrhoea, as the daily stool weight of a healthy person rarely exceeds 200 g. The profound degree of steatorrhoea strongly suggests pancreatic exocrine deficiency, rather than any of the non-pancreatic causes of steatorrhoea.

2 Assessment of fat soluble vitamin deficiency
Vitamin D and vitamin K deficiencies are commonly found in patients with steatorrhoea. Although vitamin D metabolites can be measured, the best screening test for osteomalacia is the serum alkaline phosphatase: the patient's normal alkaline phosphatase makes this diagnosis unlikely, although the definitive investigation is a bone biopsy. Vitamin K deficiency was confirmed by a prolonged pro-thrombin time (21 seconds with a control of 13 seconds) which became

normal 24 hours after vitamin K 10 mg im Vitamin A and E deficiencies are extremely rare.

3 Jejunal biopsy and aspirate of duodenal contents

The jejunal mucosa was normal, with no evidence of coeliac disease. *Giardia lamblia* could not be seen either on histological examination of the jejunal biopsy or in the aspirated duodenal juice.

4 Plain X-ray of abdomen

There was patchy calcification across the upper abdomen indicating pancreatic calcification. The appearance strongly suggested chronic calcific pancreatitis.

5 Barium small bowel meal

The whole of the small intestine appeared normal. There was neither evidence of mucosal disease affecting the small intestine, nor causes for stagnation that would allow bacterial overgrowth. There were no strictures suggesting intestinal tuberculosis or Crohn's disease.

6 Endoscopic retrograde cholangio-pancreatography (ERCP)

Gross changes of chronic calcific pancreatitis were shown affecting the whole of the pancreas. The biliary tree was normal. Cholelithiasis was excluded as a cause of the pancreatic disease.

7 A test of pancreatic exocrine function

The calcification seen in the plain X-ray of the upper abdomen, the abnormal ERCP and the demonstration of profound steatorrhoea were probably sufficient evidence that this patient had a damaged pancreas. However, either a Lundh test or a secretin-pancreozymin test could be performed to demonstrate that the damaged pancreas does not secrete digestive enzymes.

WHAT IS THE FINAL DIAGNOSIS?

Idiopathic chronic calcific pancreatitis, causing steatorrhoea and diabetes mellitus.

HOW WOULD YOU MANAGE THIS PATIENT?

Pancreatic exocrine deficiency is managed by the restriction of dietary fat intake, but it is not necessary for a patient to have an intolerable fat-free diet. Pancreatic enzyme supplements are given with every meal and with every snack between meals. However, gastric acid tends to destroy the enzyme supplements as they pass through the stomach. This destruction can sometimes be reduced by cimetidine 200 mg three times a day before meals, or less conveniently by high doses of antacids taken with every meal. As a degree of steatorrhoea will probably persist despite this treatment, the patient should be reviewed regularly to ensure that fat soluble vitamin deficiency does not develop.

Diabetes mellitus should be controlled by a restricted carbohydrate diet. Despite the absence of ketosis it is probable that only poor control will be achieved by using an oral hypoglycaemic drug. The patient will probably need insulin.

Fortunately the patient's chronic pancreatitis caused little pain. Control of pain in these patients is most unsatisfactory, many of them becoming addicted to narcotics. Sub-lingual buphrenorphine 0.4 mg six to eight-hourly may provide adequate relief of pancreatic chronic pain without the risk of addiction. Some patients are helped by coeliac ganglion blockade. Pancreatic resection is probably best restricted to those patients who are neither alcoholics nor narcotic addicts, but who have unbearable chronic pain.

COMMENT

Chronic calcific pancreatitis is unusual except in alcoholics. Calcific pancreatitis occurs in patients from the Indian subcontinent but is usually associated with malnutrition. Although the patient did give a history of chronic but mild abdominal pain, her worst episode of pain occurred after the retrograde pancreatography. After starting pancreatic enzyme supplements and restricting her fat intake the patient's steatorrhoea improved dramatically.

EXAMINERS' FOLLOW-UP QUESTIONS

1　Why did the patient lose so much weight?
2　Would abdominal ultrasound be of any help?
3　What oral hypoglycaemic drug would you recommend?
4　If that oral drug failed to control the diabetes, what type of insulin would you recommend?
5　What pancreatic enzyme supplement would you prescribe?

R.E.P.

A fat boy

WHAT IS THE DIFFERENTIAL DIAGNOSIS?

1 Prolactin secreting pituitary tumour
   Hypogonadism
   Hypothyroidism
   Hyperprolactinaemia
2 Hypothyroidism
   Delayed puberty
   Hyperprolactinaemia

The patient has failed to develop secondary sexual characteristics, and the slowed reflexes suggest that he is hypothyroid. He has gynaecomastia and galactorrhoea from the left breast, suggesting that he has hyperprolactinaemia.

The two possibilities are that he either has a prolactin-secreting pituitary tumour with secondary failure of thyroid stimulating hormone secretion, or alternatively he has primary thyroid failure, which has delayed puberty and has been associated with secondary hyperprolactinaemia.

WHAT ADDITIONAL INVESTIGATIONS WOULD YOU CONSIDER?

1 Serum prolactin concentration

This patient's serum prolactin was 8200 μU/l (normal less than 400 μU/l). This marked elevation of serum prolactin is almost certainly due to a prolactin secreting tumour. Smaller increases are seen in acromegaly or in primary myxoedema.

2 Serum thyroxine

The patient's serum thyroxine was 45 nmol/l with a free thyroxine index of 39 (normal ranges, 58–128 nmol/l and 52–142, respectively). He is hypothyroid, but thyrotropin (TSH) is not detectable. This combination suggests pituitary insufficiency, rather than failure of the thyroid gland (primary myxoedema).

3 Skull X-rays

Skull X-rays, with coned views of the sella turcica, showed marked enlargement of the pituitary fossa, with an erosion of the floor and expansion into the sphenoid space.

4 X-ray of hands and elbow

The patient's bone age was 15 years, despite his true age of 18 years.

5 Perimetry to assess visual fields

A bitemporal contraction of the visual fields is typical of an enlarging pituitary tumour, which compresses the optic chiasma. This patient did not have any abnormality of vision.

6 CT brain scan

Despite the abnormal skull X-ray, this investigation is necessary to determine whether there is a suprasellar extension of the tumour. This patient's scan suggested growth above the sella, in the region of the third ventricle.

7 Tests of pituitary reserve

An insulin stress test demonstrates the response of growth hormone and plasma cortisol to insulin-induced hypoglycaemia. The responses of both hormones were absent in this patient.

Thyrotropin releasing hormone (TRH 200 μg iv) normally causes release of thyroid stimulating hormone. This patient failed to produce a normal increase in response to TRH.

Injection of gonadotropin releasing hormone failed to stimulate release of luteinising and follicle-stimulating hormones.

These three tests demonstrate that the prolactinoma has eliminated all the normal functions of the anterior pituitary.

WHAT IS THE FINAL DIAGNOSIS?

Panhypopituitarism, due to a large prolactinoma with suprasellar extension.

HOW WOULD YOU MANAGE THIS PATIENT?

The treatment for any large pituitary tumour which has a suprasellar extension is surgical excision. This ensures the removal of the tumour and the prevention of further clinical features due to local pressure. There have been some reports of successful treatment of large prolactinomas with bromocriptine or other dopamine agonists, but this is not an established approach for the treatment of very large pressure-producing tumours. Since most tumours shrink in size following bromocriptine, it is worth treating patients with this drug if surgery is contraindicated or if it has to be postponed for some reason.

Following surgical excision, total endocrine assessment of the patient must be undertaken again. An elevated prolactin concentration indicates the presence of residual tumour, and treatment with bromocriptine or a similar agent should be commenced. This boy will need replacement therapy with cortisol, thyroxine and testosterone.

COMMENT

Large prolactinomas in young males are unusual, as is the presentation of this tumour with hypopituitarism. The failure of this boy to achieve secondary sexual development indicates that the tumour had attained a sufficient size to compress the remaining pituitary, even at the age of 12 years. Men with a prolactinoma tend to present with lack of libido, impotence and gynaecomastia. Galactorrhoea is rare.

In a female, a prolactinoma usually presents with infertility, amenorrhoea, lack of libido and galactorrhoea.

EXAMINERS' FOLLOW-UP QUESTIONS

1 Why was his bone age 15, but his chronological age 18?
2 Why did this patient not develop diabetes insipidus, either before or after the hypophysectomy?
3 Would pneumo-encephalography have been of any help in the preoperative assessment?
4 Will this patient require mineralocorticoid supplements?
5 How is replacement testosterone therapy usually administered in these patients?

P.D.

Early exhaustion

WHAT IS THE DIFFERENTIAL DIAGNOSIS?

1 Anaemia
    Malabsorption of vitamin B12 or folic acid
    Haemolytic anaemia
    Lymphoma
2 Jaundice
    Liver disease
    Pernicious anaemia
    Lymphoma
    Haemolytic anaemia

He shows many of the classical features of a severe anaemia, including angina on exertion, which is common in the elderly and is often the presenting complaint. A sore tongue may be reported in any deficiency anaemia, although it is commoner in vitamin B12 deficiency. A primary haemolytic process cannot be excluded on the information available so far; he was jaundiced, the spleen was enlarged and the high MCV could reflect a raised reticulocyte count (it would need to be over 50 per cent). An intraabdominal lymphoma is a very definite possibility with weight-loss in a man of this age; a secondary haemolytic anaemia occurs in at least 10 per cent of patients with lymphoproliferative disorders. However, the normal liver function tests would be rather unusual if there was liver involvement by lymphoma and this also makes alcohol-related liver disease less likely.

WHAT ADDITIONAL INVESTIGATIONS WOULD YOU CONSIDER?

1 Examination of blood film and reticulocyte count
The red cells showed gross anisopoikilocytosis and oval macrocytes. Many of the neutrophils were hypersegmented and the platelets were reduced on the film (platelet count $40 \times 10^9/l$). The reticulocyte count was two per cent; a haemolytic anaemia can be excluded but lymphoma still remains a possibility.

2 Bone marrow
A hypercellular sample which showed gross megaloblastic haemopoiesis, with a megaloblastic erythroid hyperplasia, and many giant metamyelocytes. There was no evidence of a lymphomatous infiltration. Although the peripheral blood and bone marrow changes

establish the diagnosis of a megaloblastic process, one needs to define the nature of the deficiency. Iron was present in abundance.

3 Vitamin B12 and folate concentrations
Serum vitamin B12: 40 ng/l (normal: 160–925 ng/l)
Serum folate: 5.4 μg/l (normal: 3–20 μg/l)
Red cell folate: 196 μg/l (normal: 160–750 μg/l)

The morphological findings and the low serum B12 value establish a diagnosis of a vitamin B12-deficient macrocytic anaemia. The cause for this deficiency needs to be investigated. Up to two months ago his appetite had been quite normal and his diet adequate. Likewise his bowel habits had been unremarkable.

4 Hydroxybutyrate dehydrogenase
This patient's hydroxybutyrate dehydrogenase concentration was 2288 IU/l (normal 70–230 IU/l). Elevated serum levels of this enzyme, a raise serum bilirubin and increased urinary urobilinogen are all seen in the typical patient with severe megaloblastic anaemia; the highest levels are seen in the most anaemic patients. Hydroxybutyrate dehydrogenase is found in bone marrow erythroid precursor cells, and is released as the great majority of these precursors die in the marrow, so-called intramedullary death or ineffective erythropoeieisis.

5 Plasma iron and total iron binding capacity
Iron: 31.8 μmol/l (normal: 15–30 μmol/l)
TIBC: 37.7 μmol/l (normal: 40–70 μmol/l)

Not a very helpful investigation. The high plasma iron and saturation level of the iron binding protein are characteristically seen in severe B12 deficiency: these levels reflect increased plasma and marrow iron turnover due to ineffective erythropoiesis. The plasma iron falls within 24 hours of starting treatment.

6 Pentagastrin test
The resting specimen of gastric juice had a pH of 7.0. After 0.6 mg pentagastrin subcutaneously the lowest pH during the next hour was 6.0 and the volume of gastric aspirate was very small. The patient has achlorhydria.

An easier way to demonstrate achlorhydria is to get the patient to eat a full breakfast early in the morning, and then fast until the late morning: a nasogastric tube is then passed to aspirate an aliquot of gastric contents. In normal people there will be plenty of acid (pH 1–3), whereas in patients with pernicious anaemia the pH will be greater than 6.

7 Schilling test

Part I: 3.1 per cent (normal: 10–25 per cent)
Part II (with added intrinsic factor): 14.7 per cent (normal: 10–25 per cent)

This result gives a clear distinction with substantial improvement with added intrinsic factor; it is diagnostic of pernicious anaemia. Sometimes, the Part II result may be low, suggesting intestinal malabsorption. Two explanations are possible: either there is impaired ileal uptake of B12 following the prolonged B12 deficiency, or intrinsic factor antibodies are present which inhibit the B12 absorption.

The Schilling test has become the most widely-used test for vitamin B12 absorption. There is no need to perform this with any urgency as the gastric lesion is not going to change. Indeed, delaying the test for a few weeks after treatment with vitamin B12 may allow the ileal mucosa to recover. The popular Dicopac test, which performs both parts of the Schilling test at the same time, is unreliable even though it is convenient.

8 Antibody tests

Gastric parietal cell: strongly positive
Intrinsic factor: negative

Parietal cell antibody is found in the serum of more than 90 per cent of patients with pernicious anaemia. The frequency of parietal cell antibodies in the adult general population is between five and eight per cent.

An antibody to intrinsic factor is detected in the serum of just over half the patients with pernicious anaemia. There are two types of intrinsic factor antibody: type I. the blocking antibody which prevents vitamin B12 binding to intrinsic factor; type II. the binding or precipitating antibody which reacts with intrinsic factor or with the intrinsic factor-vitamin B12 complex. The type I antibody occurs in about 55 per cent of patients, and type II in 35 per cent. 45 per cent of patients show no antibody to intrinsic factor.

9 Upper gastrointestinal endoscopy

'The oesophagus is normal; the mucosa of the stomach is very pale, but no lesion is seen. The duodenal mucosa is normal. Gastric mucosal biopsies taken.'

The histology report was as follows: 'The gastric mucosa and submucosa show intestinal metaplasia. The appearances are those of chronic non-specific gastritis.'

This patient was gastroscoped because of his symptoms of anorexia and weight loss. In the absence of symptoms a gastroscopy is not warranted nor is a barium meal necessary, although many physicians arrange these tests when pernicious anaemia is diagnosed. The risk of gastric malignancy in a patient with pernicious anaemia is only increased three-fold when compared with the general population.

WHAT IS THE FINAL DIAGNOSIS?

Pernicious anaemia.

HOW WOULD YOU MANAGE THIS PATIENT?

The patient should be given parenteral vitamin B12 (hydroxocobalamin) for life. There are no hard rules defining how much needs to be given but, in the severely anaemic patient, 1 mg (1000 μg) hydroxocobalamin can be given daily by injection for a week; sufficient will be retained to replenish the B12 stores. The benefit from therapy is rapid. The severely anaemic patient will notice a non-specific improvement in 24-48 hours, and a reticulocyte peak appears in about seven days. The long-term maintenance therapy needs to supply 5 μg vitamin B12 daily; this is achieved by giving 1 mg every two or three months.

The use of blood transfusions in patients with severe anaemia should be avoided; many are in incipient heart failure, and the cardiac muscle is ill-equipped to increase its work-load after many months of severe anaemia.

The need to give potassium supplements is not proven, but it has been suggested that the rapid movement of potassium into newly-formed cells may lead to hypokalaemia; perhaps the best that can be said is that the serum potassium concentration should be measured regularly in the severely anaemic patient. Folate supplements are rarely required: when the patient feels better a good diet will provide adequate folate. Iron supplements are quite often required in the later stages of the haemopoietic recovery and ferrous sulphate 200-400 mg daily will be adequate, and should be prescribed for three months.

COMMENT

With increasing age the prevalence of pernicious anaemia increases, but it can occur even in childhood. Long-term follow-up should be carried out by the patient's general practitioner. An annual blood count is recommended. Any dyspepsia should be investigated, as these patients never get peptic ulceration. It is impracticable to look for the early development of a gastric carcinoma by performing an annual barium meal or gastroscopy.

It is often the practice to give both vitamin B12 and folic acid to patients with a macrocytic megaloblastic anaemia until the results of the assays are available. The only justification for this practice is in the severely anaemic and ill patient. Occasionally megaloblastic patients present with bleeding due to severe thrombocytopenia, and they should always be given both vitamin B12 and folic acid immediately.

EXAMINERS' FOLLOW-UP QUESTIONS

1 What causes atrophic gastritis?
2 What are the signs of sub-acute combined degeneration of the spinal cord?
3 Name reasons for vitamin B12 malabsorption, other than pernicious anaemia.
4 What group of British patients may have a nutritional B12 deficiency?
5 How do you perform a pentagastrin test?

E.J.P.-W.

Bloody diarrhoea

WHAT IS THE DIFFERENTIAL DIAGNOSIS?

1   Ulcerative colitis
    Crohn's disease of the colon
    Colitis, due to infection
      Clostridium difficile
      Campylobacter jejuni
      Salmonella
      Shigella
      Amoebiasis

Diverticular disease of the colon may cause a brisk haemorrhage, and
it may cause diarrhoea, but it almost never causes prolonged bloody
diarrhoea. Although the patient had no definite history of inflammatory bowel disease, the bowel upset two years earlier could have
been a milder episode of the same illness. Several infectious causes of
colitis are also quite possible in this patient: pseudomembranous
colitis could have been induced by the course of ampicillin; the patient
is single and enteric infections are much more common in male
homosexuals, but the patient denied homosexual activity.

WHAT ADDITIONAL INVESTIGATIONS WOULD YOU CONSIDER?

1   Sigmoidoscopy and rectal biopsy
Early sigmoidoscopy is mandatory in a patient who is hospitalised with
bloody diarrhoea. The patient's rectum contained blood and pus: there
was spontaneous ulceration and friability of the mucosa. These
changes are seen in any acute colitis, and a biopsy should always be
taken. Urgent histology confirmed a non-specific colitis, but no
granulomata were observed. This makes Crohn's disease less likely,
but does not exclude it. It is usually impossible for the histologist to
differentiate confidently an infectious colitis from ulcerative colitis.

2   Stools for parasites, culture and *Cl. difficile* toxin
It is imperative that stools are urgently examined to exclude all the
likely infections. To avoid delay, it is often best for the
sigmoidoscopist, at the time of the admission sigmoidoscopy, to collect
the first stool specimen. This patient's stools contained no pathogens,
but the patient was kept in 'enteric isolation' until they were reported
to be pathogen-free, which took 48 hours.

3 Supine plain X-ray of the abdomen

Faeces were observed in the caecum and descending colon, but gas-filled bowel extended from the mid-transverse colon, down the left side, to the rectum. The bowel was not dilated (that is, it was less than 6 cm at its widest point), and no sloughing of the mucosa ('mucosal islands') was visible. The length of gas-filled bowel reveals the extent of inflamed colonic mucosa, and the degree of dilatation provides a warning of impending perforation.

4 Barium enema X-ray

A barium enema in a patient with fulminant colitis is hazardous; the plain film provides quite sufficient information to manage the patient. A barium enema should be delayed until the patient has recovered.

5 Four-hourly temperature and pulse, stool chart

A fever greater than 38°C or frequent bowel actions (eight per 24 hours) during the day after admission have been shown to carry a poor prognosis for patients with acute colitis. In the 24 hours after admission, this patient had a maximum temperature of 38.2°C and opened his bowels nine times. He also displayed two of three other 'high risk for colectomy' features: a low serum albumin and oral thrush. Although mucosal islands, the fifth bad feature, were not seen in this patient's plain abdominal X-rays, he was undoubtedly very ill and was likely to require an early colectomy, unless he made a dramatic recovery.

WHAT IS THE FINAL DIAGNOSIS?

Severe ulcerative colitis.

HOW WOULD YOU MANAGE THIS PATIENT?

The patient is extremely catabolic but anorexic. He should receive total parenteral nutrition if he does not feel like eating. He is anaemic and should receive an immediate four-unit blood transfusion to raise his haemoglobin from 8.2 to 12.0 g/dl. He should be rested in bed, and provided with sufficient oral fluids to keep him comfortable. The oral thrush should be treated with topical nystatin or amphotericin B.

It may take up to 48 hours after admission for investigations to eliminate the infectious causes of colitis. If possible steroids should be delayed until the results of these tests are available. If they are negative, the patient should then receive intravenous prednisolone: 32 mg twice a day. The patient has an iritis and should receive steroid eye drops.

A surgeon should be consulted immediately after admission, and joint consultations should take place every day. Progress can be assessed using stool and temperature/pulse charts, but particularly by daily supine abdominal X-ray films. Early deterioration, particularly with increasing colonic dilatation on the plain X-rays, or continuing illness after five days of intensive treatment, would encourage an emergency colectomy.

If the patient improves after five days, he may change to oral prednisolone, and oral sulphasalazine 1 g bd may be added. Sulphasalazine maintenance treatment at this dose undoubtedly reduces the incidence of relapse.

COMMENT

The management of acute ulcerative colitis demands much attention to detail, complete confidence between physician and surgeon, and experience. Unnecessary colectomy is a disaster, but inadvertent perforation of the colon carries a mortality of approximately 30 per cent.

Whenever a patient presents with colitis, whether the first attack or a mild relapse in an out-patient, the stools must always be reexamined for infection. Any infection is treated by specific therapy, and steroids avoided.

This patient made a full recovery. His colitis remained in remission for nine months until, against medical advice, he stopped sulphasalazine maintenance treatment.

EXAMINERS' FOLLOW-UP QUESTIONS

1 When would you use rectal corticosteroids, and what preparations are available?
2 What do you know about mesalazine (5-aminosalicylic acid)?
3 What is the difference between *Salmonella* colitis, and typhoid fever?
4 Does sodium cromoglycate help patients with inflammatory bowel disease?
5 What are the side-effects of sulphasalazine?

R.E.P.

Sickle cell anaemia

WHAT IS THE DIFFERENTIAL DIAGNOSIS?

1   Sickle cell anaemia
       Painful bone crisis
       Aplastic crisis
2   Acute pulmonary episode
       Pneumonia
       Pulmonary infarction
       Bone marrow embolism

The illness started with an upper respiratory tract infection: she sought advice from her family doctor, who correctly put her on a broad-spectrum antibiotic. The subsequent development of bone pain in different sites is a common event after an infection, which disturbs the normal steady-state of sickle cell anaemia. The pain was not severe but it did require simple analgesics. The anaemia may be due to a number of causes, but it is worth noting that she is not jaundiced. This is unusual in sickle cell anaemia and suggests red cell aplasia. Despite being on antibiotics, the patient became desperately ill with a severe respiratory problem.

WHAT ADDITIONAL INVESTIGATIONS WOULD YOU CONSIDER?

1   Blood film
Very few sickled cells were seen on examination of the blood film, and no polychromatic red cells or nucleated red cells were present. The number of sickled cells varies between patients, but in an individual patient it is fairly constant. The absence of polychromatic cells, and a degree of anaemia more severe than expected, together with a normal bilirubin concentration, are most likely to be due to impaired red cell production.

2   Reticulocyte count
0.1 per cent. For someone with a severe haemolytic anaemia this was a surprisingly low value (usually 5–30 per cent in sickle cell anaemia). Two possibilities are likely: folic acid deficiency or a red cell aplastic crisis. She was known to be an irregular taker of folic acid, but a bone marrow examination would resolve this issue very quickly.

3   Bone marrow examination
A moderately cellular marrow was obtained, with a reduced granulocyte/erythroid ratio of 2:1 (normal 4:1 to 7:1). This abnormal ratio is due to an excess of red cell precursors: in sickle cell anaemia

there is usually an erythroid hyperplasia with 50–70 per cent of the marrow cells being erythroblasts. Erythropoiesis was normoblastic, but all the erythroid cells were early normoblasts and no mature forms were present. There were no megaloblastic changes suggesting folic acid deficiency. This 'maturation arrest' in the erythroid development is characteristic of the recovery phase of an aplastic crisis, which was probably induced by the respiratory infection. If blood counts are done regularly at this stage, one would expect a 'flood' of normoblasts and reticulocytes in the peripheral blood over the next few days.

4   Chest radiograph
There were changes consistent with consolidation of the right lower lobe. The clinical features of acute onset, fever, leucocytosis and severe dyspnoea are more likely to be due to infection than to a pulmonary-vascular occlusion.

5   Blood culture
No growth, but she had been started on antibiotics before these cultures were taken. Causal organisms are isolated in only half of the acute, febrile pulmonary episodes in sickle cell anaemia. As this patient could produce no sputum, and a bacteraemia occurs in many patients with pneumonia, it would be worthwhile trying to isolate an organism in a blood culture.

6   Blood gases
pH: 7.2 (normal: 7.35–7.45)
PCO_2: 3.3 kPa (normal: 4.5–6.0 kPa)
PO_2: 8.1 kPa (normal: 12–15 kPa)
Base excess: 15.3 mmol/l (normal: − 2.0–2.0 mmol/l)
Standard bicarbonate 12.5 mmol/l (normal: 21.0–25.0 mmol/l)
These figures were obtained whilst breathing 40 per cent oxygen. She was profoundly ill, with dyspnoea and tachypnoea exceeding the amount of lung pathology evident from the chest radiograph. In the acute infectious pulmonary episodes of sickle cell anaemia, a lowered arterial oxygen saturation is often encountered. A number of factors may contribute to this, such as decreased membrane diffusing capacity, an increased pulmonary-capillary blood volume, and an increased shunting of mixed-venous blood through the lungs.

7   Lung scan
No under-perfused areas were demonstrated. If there is any doubt as to whether the lung pathology is infective or due to infarction, a lung scan can be helpful. In sickle cell disease the vascular lesions are usually microthrombotic, but patchy perfusion defects may be observed.

WHAT IS THE FINAL DIAGNOSIS?

Sickle cell anaemia, with lobar pneumonia and an associated aplastic red cell crisis.

HOW WOULD YOU MANAGE THIS PATIENT?

This is a complicated patient who has a number of different problems occurring simultaneously; all are interacting to her detriment. She has a serious infective pulmonary sickle cell crisis.

Prompt treatment should be started with intravenous benzyl penicillin and gentamicin, and continuous '100 per cent' oxygen therapy. The blood gases should be measured at frequent intervals. She should receive an immediate partial exchange transfusion. Two units of blood (1000 ml) are removed, giving 500 ml 0.9% saline between the two 'donations', and then infusing 5 units of packed red cells. Because of her severe, aregenerative anaemia, removal of the first 500 ml of blood would probably suffice. This will reduce endogenous red cell production and so keep the percentage of haemoglobin S below 30 per cent. Oral alkalinising drugs are not recommended — it is doubtful if they help.

Any patient with sickle cell anaemia is very sensitive to fluid deprivation: it is most important to maintain hydration, especially during a febrile crisis.

COMMENT

At any age, sickle cell anaemia patients are very prone to infections, particularly in the respiratory tract. The non-functioning spleen and defects in the alternate complement pathway make them particularly susceptible to *Pneumococcal* infections. Aplastic red cell crises are frequently precipitated by infection, particularly with parvovirus, and are recognised by the severe anaemia and a very low reticulocyte count. They are self-limiting episodes and spontaneous recovery is the rule, but blood transfusion support may be necessary.

The major difficulty in diagnosing an acute pulmonary episode in sickle cell disease is deciding whether the illness is due to bacterial infection, pulmonary infarction, or both. It is probably wise to treat all these pulmonary episodes as infective, and if there is only slow resolution after appropriate antibiotic therapy, an underlying pulmonary infarction should be considered. A positive lung scan would indicate the need for intravenous heparin therapy, followed by oral anticoagulant therapy for three months. Cardiac failure may further complicate an already difficult problem.

Polyvalent *Pneumococcal* vaccine should be given to all patients with sickle cell anaemia, but there are many occasions when this fails to protect against a subtype not offered in the vaccine. Oral penicillin

V 250 mg bd is strongly advocated, probably for life, although good compliance is unlikely. The greatest mortality rate for patients with sickle cell disease is in the first three years. Survivors still have a shortened life expectancy, but many live long enough to have children.

EXAMINERS' FOLLOW-UP QUESTIONS

1 What contraceptive advice would you give this girl?
2 How would you approach the question of genetic counselling for someone with sickle cell disease?
3 What is haemoglobin SC disease?
4 Why did this patient's admission urine contain red cells?
5 What bone changes will be seen in this patient's X-rays?

E.J.P.-W.

Post-operative confusion

WHAT IS THE DIFFERENTIAL DIAGNOSIS?

1 Hyponatraemia with convulsions
2 Cerebrovascular accident
3 Gram negative septicaemia
4 Inappropriate anti-diuretic hormone (ADH) syndrome
5 Congestive cardiac failure
6 Silent myocardial infarction
7 Post-operative bronchopneumonia
8 Drug-induced toxic confusional state

The very low serum sodium has developed quickly. This in itself is sufficient to produce neurological symptoms and signs due to cerebral oedema. The fall in osmolarity occurs much more rapidly in plasma than can occur within the central nervous system. There is a marked influx of water into the brain, resulting in raised intracranial pressure and cerebral oedema.

His intravenous replacement regimen consisted of three litres of dextrose-saline per day: the patient received approximately 90 mmol of sodium per day. The low urea and reduced concentrations of other plasma electrolytes suggest dilution.

In the absence of a local venous obstruction, a raised JVP with oedema means circulatory overload, and implies a degree of right-sided cardiac failure. Oedema *always* means salt *and* water overload. Although the patient undoubtedly has hyponatraemia, which is largely dilutional, additionally he is sodium-overloaded. Pure water intoxication produces neither oedema nor a raised JVP, as water diffuses freely throughout the tissues.

It is possible that the stress of major surgery could have resulted in a cerebrovascular accident. The lack of any focal neurological sign is against this diagnosis, and a careful scrutiny of his operation notes and anaesthetic charts did not reveal any period of hypotension that might lead to cerebral thrombosis.

Hypoxia and drug-induced confusional states need to be considered. In the absence of cyanosis, hypoxia can be ruled out. All sedative drugs should be withdrawn if possible.

The sodium and water handling in this patient is complicated but is best understood by discussing the physiological consequences of reduced renal perfusion. Any cause of reduced kidney perfusion (cardiac failure, hypovolaemia, nephrotic syndrome, or advanced hepatic cirrhosis) causes intense proximal and distal tubular sodium reabsorption. *Proximal* sodium reabsorption occurs because any fall in renal perfusion pressure is followed by a fall in the peritubular capillary hydrostatic pressure, which promotes avid proximal tubular sodium reabsorption. Increased *distal* tubular sodium reabsorption is due to raised aldosterone secretion. Increased amounts of antidiuretic hormone (ADH) are also released in cardiac failure, nephrotic syndrome and cirrhosis (as far as signals for ADH release are concerned, the need to preserve circulating blood volume overrides osmolarity regulation). It is therefore apparent that this patient's sodium intake could easily have exceeded his ability to excrete sodium, and this is the cause of the oedema. It is not uncommon for patients with cardiac failure, hypovolaemia, nephrotic syndrome, or cirrhosis to excrete less than 10 mmol sodium daily.

Why did this patient develop a low plasma sodium? This occurs because poorly perfused kidneys are unable to make dilute urine. This patient cannot excrete a water load, as his ability to produce 'free water' is impaired. The reason for this is tied up with the avid proximal sodium reabsorption. When there is avid proximal sodium reabsorption, there is simultaneous proximal reabsorption of water (proximal isosmotic reabsorption). This decreases the amount of solute delivered to the ascending limb of the loop of Henlé, which is the only place where sodium can be reabsorbed leaving water behind in the tubule. This is the point where 'free water' is normally generated. The ability to excrete a water load is therefore severely compromised when only a little solute reaches this part of the nephron. If water intake continues, hyponatraemia will develop. If ADH is increased, free water excretion is even further impaired.

A low plasma sodium raises the possibility of inappropriate ADH secretion. The stress of an intercurrent operation can be followed by raised ADH secretion, but this seldom produces a profound dilutional hyponatraemia such as was seen in this man. A neurological lesion occurring at the time of operation or chronic chest disease could be the stimulus to inappropriate secretion of ADH in a patient like this. Before this syndrome can be diagnosed with certainty, renal, endocrine (adrenal and thyroid), liver, and cardiac disease must be excluded. Inappropriate ADH secretion which leads to retention of water does not produce oedema.

WHAT ADDITIONAL INVESTIGATIONS WOULD YOU CONSIDER?

1 Urinary composition

The urinary sodium and osmolarity will help to define the cause of the hyponatraemia. The urinary sodium concentration was 15 mmol/l. This implies sodium retention by the kidney, and suggests that there is reduced renal perfusion. It excludes secretion of inappropriate ADH as the cause of the dilutional hyponatraemia, as the sodium concentration would be much higher. The urine osmolarity was high at 495 mosmol/kg: the patient was producing concentrated high quality urine. He was unable to produce dilute urine, which would be the normal response to water overloading.

2 Chest X-ray

The chest X-ray taken on the fourth post-operative day showed a little basal atelectasis on the right. The heart size had increased by 1 cm from a preoperative routine chest film. There was a minor degree of upper lobe venous diversion. The chest X-ray therefore confirms the presence of cardiac failure and supports the diagnosis of salt and water overload.

A silent myocardial infarction is not uncommon in the elderly. It could be partly to blame for tipping this patient into congestive cardiac failure. An ECG and cardiac enzymes would help to exclude this possibility.

3 ECG and cardiac enzymes

The ECG was abnormal. There was extensive ST depression with T wave inversion in leads I and II and well as the left chest lead. There was no evidence of a recent myocardial infarction. These changes would be compatible with a digoxin effect as well as myocardial ischaemia. The cardiac enzymes were normal.

4 Plasma osmolarity

The plasma osmolarity can be calculated from the screening results when results are expressed in SI units (mmol/l). The plasma osmolarity is equal to twice the sum of the sodium and potassium concentration, plus that of the urea and glucose. The patient's blood glucose was 3 mmol/l. In this patient this gives a calculated plasma osmolarity of 230 which slightly underestimates the measured value of 239 mosmol/kg. An osmolarity as low as this, if it develops quickly, is sufficient to produce the cerebral oedema and neurological features that this patient developed. The normal plasma osmolarity is approximately 285 mosmol/kg.

5 Bacteriology

Operations on the biliary tract are commonly complicated by sepsis. The absence of shock, fever and the normal white cell count are against a septicaemia. Blood and urine cultures should, however, be carried out just to make sure that infection is not missed.

WHAT IS THE FINAL DIAGNOSIS?

Hyponatraemia with cerebral oedema, due to inappropriate fluid replacement and reduced 'free water' clearance. Mild congestive cardiac failure was caused by ischaemic heart disease.

HOW WOULD YOU MANAGE THIS PATIENT?

Rapidly-developing hyponatraemia with neurological signs has a bad prognosis. As this causes death in up to 50 per cent of these patients, treatment has to be carried out promptly and effectively.

In most cases a dilutional hyponatraemia will resolve by restricting the patient's access to water. This patient's intravenous infusion should be stopped and he should be given mouth washes only.

To reduce the cerebral oedema, it is necessary to raise the plasma osmolarity. In the absence of fluid overload and cardiac failure this can be achieved readily by infusing 100 ml 20 per cent mannitol over one to two hours. Mannitol acts as an osmotic diuretic, blocking sodium reabsorption in the proximal tubule. This means that more solute is presented to the diluting segment of the nephron (ascending limb of the loop of Henlé), which increases free water clearance, helping resolution of the hyponatraemia. An osmotic diuretic may be the ideal diuretic to use in this sort of clinical situation.

However, it would be extremely dangerous to use mannitol in this man, who already has an expanded intravascular volume (raised JVP) and is in cardiac failure. An infusion of mannitol would acutely expand the blood volume, and would probably precipitate pulmonary oedema.

A different approach has to be adopted in this patient. To control the cardiac failure, intravenous frusemide should be given to produce a brisk diuresis (100–150 ml/hour). In a man of this age it would be prudent to insert a urethral catheter to ensure adequate drainage and to facilitate hourly urine volume measurements.

When a good diuresis has been well-established, twice normal saline (1.8 per cent containing approximately 300 mmol/l sodium) should be infused at about 50 ml/hour. Infusion of hypertonic saline before the congestive cardiac failure has been controlled would provoke pulmonary oedema. In this way the plasma osmolarity is raised, cerebral oedema reduced, and the excess salt and water (oedema) can be mobilised. It is better to control hyponatraemia slowly over two to three days, so that rapid changes in brain cell volume can be avoided. Cerebral oedema can also be reduced by giving dexamethasone (12 mg/day), which can be reduced over the next few days (steroids are of most benefit when the cerebral oedema is due to inflammatory intracranial lesions). Fits should be treated with intravenous diazepam or chloromethiazole.

After this patient's hyponatraemia had responded to treatment, his i.v. fluid regimen was altered so that he was receiving one litre of normal saline together with 500 ml of 5 per cent dextrose. He was given in addition a total of 80 mmol of potassium/24 hours, in divided doses added to the infusion bags. He made a full recovery with no evidence of permanent neurological damage.

COMMENT

Hyponatraemia is life-threatening if it develops quickly and is severe. The diagnostic approach is based on recognising in which of the three major groups a hyponatraemic patient properly resides:

1 Loss of more sodium than water

This is true sodium depletion and is relatively uncommon. There should therefore be good clinical evidence of a low total body sodium: there should be evidence of contraction of the extracellular fluid volume. This is manifest by postural hypotension, reduced tissue turgor, empty veins and perhaps poor peripheral perfusion. Adrenal insufficiency or a salt-losing nephritis can cause this clinical problem.

2 Retention of water only

Pure water intoxication does not produce peripheral oedema as the water is freely diffusable throughout all compartments and within cells. The intracellular compartment is expanded together with a much more modest expansion of the extracellular fluid volume. Inappropriate ADH secretion causes this type of problem. Other causes include compulsive water drinking and inappropriate fluid therapy with either 5% dextrose or dextrose-saline.

3 Retention of relatively more water than sodium

This is the commonest group of patients with hyponatraemia. There is retention of sodium but there is an even greater retention of water. This group should be subdivided into those with evidence of an expanded intravascular volume (eg cardiac failure), and those with evidence of a reduced effective circulating blood volume (eg the nephrotic syndrome or advanced cirrhosis). In both of the subtypes of group 3 there is retention of sodium, and there is therefore oedema.

EXAMINERS' FOLLOW-UP QUESTIONS

1 What are the causes of inappropriate secretion of ADH?
2 What drugs affect ADH secretion?
3 Is digoxin of any benefit for a patient with heart failure, who is in sinus rhythm?
4 What causes of salt depletion do you know?
5 If you had been asked to see this patient pre-operatively, what fluid and diuretic regimens would you have recommended?

P.S.

Progressive jaundice

WHAT IS THE DIFFERENTIAL DIAGNOSIS?

1 Carcinoma of the head of the pancreas
  Carcinoma of the bile duct
2 Diabetes mellitus

The combination of progressive cholestatic jaundice, with recent onset of diabetes, in an elderly man strongly suggests the diagnosis of carcinoma of the pancreas. The possibly enlarged gall-bladder supports the diagnosis.

Carcinoma of the bile ducts at the hilum of the liver is a possibility, but this would not explain either the diabetes or the palpable gall-bladder.

WHAT ADDITIONAL INVESTIGATIONS WOULD YOU CONSIDER?

1 Examination of the faeces
The appearance was silvery due to a combination of steatorrhoea and melaena. This would support a diagnosis of pancreatic carcinoma. Occult blood tests on the faeces were consistently positive.

2 Urine tests
The urine showed absence of urobilinogen on five consecutive days. In a patient with cholestasis this strongly supports total biliary obstruction and pancreatic cancer becomes a strong possibility.

3 Prothrombin time
This was 20 seconds with a control value of 13 seconds. After 10 mg vitamin K1 intramuscularly for two days the prothrombin time was 15 seconds with a control of 13 seconds. Restoration of the prothrombin time with vitamin K implies that hepatocellular function is adequate for prothrombin synthesis and supports the diagnosis of cholestatic jaundice.

4 Ultrasound
This showed markedly dilated bile ducts within the liver. The common bile duct also seemed to be dilated. The gall-bladder was enlarged, but stones were not seen in it. The pancreatic duct was dilated.

These findings support an obstruction at the lower end of the common bile duct involving the pancreatic duct; carcinoma must be the most likely possibility.

5 Barium meal

Showed a deformity in the medial aspect of the second part of the duodenum which resembled a reversed number 3. The duodenal loop was enlarged. These findings suggest a large tumour in the head of the pancreas with possible duodenal invasion.

6 Chest X-ray

This was done to exclude pulmonary metastases. The chest X-ray was normal, apart from a raised right diaphragm presumably due to an enlarged liver.

7 CT scan of the abdomen

This was not in fact performed on this patient, as the less costly ultrasound and barium meal had shown a large pancreatic mass which was presumably malignant. CT scanning however, is very useful in visualising lesions on the posterior abdominal wall and would show dilated intrahepatic and common bile ducts, and the gall-bladder. It could have replaced ultrasound in this patient.

WHAT IS THE FINAL DIAGNOSIS?

Carcinoma of the head of the pancreas, causing diabetes mellitus and biliary obstruction.

HOW WOULD YOU MANAGE THIS PATIENT?

Vitamin K1 10 mg intramuscularly is given daily. A low-fat diet is given in as attractive a form as possible. The most obvious course would be to refer the patient immediately for bypass surgery, usually a choledocho-jejunostomy, or cholecysto-enterostomy. The first procedure is preferable as the anastomosis remains patent even if the cystic duct becomes obstructed. Either procedure would relieve both the jaundice and the pruritus. At surgery, the pancreatic tumour was large and invading adjacent structures, including the splenic vein, so that resection was not possible. A biopsy from the tumour was performed and showed adenocarcinoma. A choledocho-jejunostomy with an entero-entero anastomosis was duly performed. In addition, a gastro-enterostomy was done, so that if duodenal obstruction developed later it would be relieved. The post-operative course was uneventful and the patient was discharged from hospital two weeks post-operatively.

The insertion of an endoprosthesis trans-hepatically or via an endoscope was considered. This would have avoided a surgical exploration and a general anaesthetic, but it would not have permitted operability to be assessed, and the gastro-enterostomy could not have been performed. In older, poor risk patients the non-surgical approach is being used increasingly.

COMMENT

Painless obstructive jaundice in an elderly patient always suggests carcinoma of the head of the pancreas. The possibility of surgical excision is very remote and a biliary-intestinal bypass operation is the standard method of management.

Patients may be unsuitable for surgery on account of such features as advanced age, other serious diseases, metastases, or a very large pancreatic tumour diagnosed pre-operatively. For these patients the insertion of an endoprosthesis (either percutaneous trans-hepatic or endoscopically) through the growth into the duodenum has revolutionised management. These techniques, however, are specialised and are not available in every hospital.

An attempt should always be made to get a tissue diagnosis: percutaneous fine-needle aspiration of a pancreatic mass sometimes provides adequate cytological or histological material. The aspiration can be guided either by ultrasound or a CT scan of the abdomen.

EXAMINERS' FOLLOW-UP QUESTIONS

1 Give the likely prognosis for this patient.
2 How would you control pain if it developed?
3 Why did this patient have no urobilinogen in his urine?
4 Why did this patient have steatorrhoea?
5 Give five possible abnormal findings on the skin of a patient with carcinoma of the pancreas.

S.S.

Diarrhoea and abdominal pain

WHAT IS THE DIFFERENTIAL DIAGNOSIS?

1   Crohn's disease
    Ulcerative colitis
    Intestinal tuberculosis
    Amoebiasis
    Antibiotic-associated (*Clostridium difficile*) colitis
    Yersinia enterocolitis

The combination of an acute illness, with weight loss, anaemia, raised
ESR and low serum albumin all point to organic rather than functional
illness. The perianal skin tags and the anal fissure make Crohn's
disease more likely; the lack of a florid colitis on sigmoidoscopy makes
ulcerative colitis less likely. Infections can mimic Crohn's disease and
they must always be excluded.

WHAT ADDITIONAL INVESTIGATIONS WOULD YOU CONSIDER?

1   Rectal biopsy
If inflammatory bowel disease is suspected in a patient with diarrhoea
a rectal biopsy should always be taken even if the mucosa appears
healthy. This patient's rectal biopsy showed non-specific inflammatory changes; no granulomata were seen.

2   Stool culture and search for parasites
Salmonella, *Shigella*, and *Campylobacter* can all cause a colitis, but
are excluded by routine stool culture. Amoebiasis (particularly
relevant as this patient had travelled in Africa) is best excluded by
rapid examination of the rectal mucus rather than stool: no parasites
were detected.

3   *Cl. difficile* toxin in the stool
Pseudomembranous colitis usually follows the use of broad spectrum
antibiotics. The toxin can be detected in the stool, or the organism
cultured using selective media; both tests were negative.

4   C-reactive protein
83 ng/ml (< 5 ng/ml). C-reactive protein is an acute phase protein,
whose concentration rises when there is inflammation. The elevated
C-reactive protein confirms that the patient has an organic disease
but, like an elevated ESR, it does not localise the site of inflammation.
However, in Crohn's disease it is more sensitive than the ESR, and it is

a most useful screening test for patients with diarrhoea and abdominal pain.

4 Barium follow-through X-ray
The radiologist reported that the jejunum appeared normal, but the distal ileum was abnormal, with an irregular mucosa pattern narrowing a thickened bowel wall. The radiologist's differential diagnosis was Crohn's disease, intestinal tuberculosis, lymphoma and a Yersinia infection.

5 Yersinia antibody
The agglutination tests for Y. pseudotuberculosis and Y. enteropathica were negative. Yersinia infection is very unusual in Britain, but it is a cause of a self-limiting inflammation of the terminal ileum.

6 Double-contrast barium enema
The whole colon was displayed. It appeared normal except for an ill-defined irregularity in the transverse colon — perhaps due to a colitis or faecal contamination. Patchy disease of the colon favours the diagnosis of Crohn's colitis rather than ulcerative colitis.

7 Colonoscopy
This invasive procedure was necessary only because of the equivocal barium enema and the need for a tissue diagnosis. The colonoscopist found multiple aphthous ulcers in the transverse colon. Biopsy of these lesions revealed histology typical of Crohn's disease, with non-caseating granulomata.

WHAT IS THE FINAL DIAGNOSIS?

Crohn's disease of the terminal ileum and colon.

HOW WOULD YOU MANAGE THIS PATIENT?

Systemic steroids usually induce a dramatic improvement. Treatment may be started with prednisolone 30–40 mg/day by mouth, the dose being reduced over the following weeks.

Sulphasalazine may also be started but its main use is as long-term maintenance treatment. It is of definite benefit in patients with colonic Crohn's disease, but its usefulness is less certain when disease is limited to the small bowel. Most patients tolerate sulphasalazine 1 g bd after meals, but the drug can cause nausea, haemolysis, and a low sperm count.

Despite maintenance treatment with sulphasalazine, Crohn's disease may relapse as the oral prednisolone is gradually reduced. Some patients may only be kept in good health by taking prednisolone

7–8 mg/day. If more prednisolone is needed, azathioprine 2 mg/kg may be tried for its prednisolone-sparing effect. Azathioprine is a dangerous drug: the patient and family doctor should be warned of the symptoms of agranulocytosis. Weekly, and then monthly, full blood counts should always be performed.

Surgery is reserved for the relief of intestinal obstruction, fistulae and abscesses. 'Cosmetic' anal surgery must be avoided. Perianal sepsis is much helped by metronidazole.

A special diet is unnecessary, but any patient with small intestinal strictures may be helped by avoiding high residue lumps of food, such as the pith of citrus fruits.

This patient was anaemic: his ferritin, B12, and folate should be checked. Patients with Crohn's disease may have a deficiency of these haematinics, and they often require specific therapy.

COMMENT

If at all possible, a tissue diagnosis of Crohn's disease should always be achieved — for fear of missing tuberculosis, amoebiasis, or lymphoma. Inadvertent steroid treatment of either infection may be fatal — precise diagnosis of the latter may be less important, for even with the early diagnosis and chemotherapy the prognosis of gut lymphoma is extremely poor.

The great majority of patients with Crohn's disease lead a full and relatively healthy life. The patients most at risk are those who, in the early years of their illness, suffer from aggressive disease requiring repeated surgery.

EXAMINERS' FOLLOW-UP QUESTIONS

1. Give four renal complications of Crohn's disease.
2. How would you treat diarrhoea after resection of the terminal ileum?
3. What skin, eye and joint symptoms may be associated with Crohn's disease?
4. How is sulphasalazine thought to help patients with inflammatory bowel disease?
5. How would you treat *Campylobacter* colitis?

R.E.P.

A young stroke

WHAT IS THE DIFFERENTIAL DIAGNOSIS?

1   Arterial emboli
    Mitral leaflet prolapse
    Paradoxical embolus
    Trivial rheumatic mitral valve disease
    Intracardiac tumour (left atrial myxoma)
    Infective endocarditis

There is clinical evidence that the patient has had at least two peripheral emboli: one cerebral and one to the right leg. In addition the episode of abdominal pain may well have been due to a third embolus. In such patients a cardiac cause is frequently sought, but not usually found unless there is additional evidence of heart disease. This patient had a transient late systolic murmur, and in addition she has an elevated ESR and a normocytic, normochromic anaemia. These abnormalities raise the possibility of a systemic disease.

WHAT ADDITIONAL INVESTIGATIONS WOULD YOU CONSIDER?

1   Blood cultures
Three blood cultures were sterile.

2   Chest X-ray and ECG
Both were normal.

3   Echocardiography
An M-mode echocardiogram showed a large left atrial myxoma behind the anterior cusp of the mitral valve. The tumour was confirmed by two-dimensional echocardiography, which demonstrated that it was approximately 3 cm across and was attached to the inter-atrial septum. The right side of the heart was normal.

WHAT IS THE FINAL DIAGNOSIS?

Multiple systemic emboli from a left atrial myoxma.

HOW WOULD YOU MANAGE THIS PATIENT?

The only treatment for a left atrial myxoma is early surgery. This should be performed within 24 hours unless there are contra-indications. In this patient, a recent cerebral embolism led to the operation being delayed for one week, since cardio-pulmonary bypass requires that the patient is heparinised.

The risk of the operation itself is low, although there may be a transient increase in the severity of any central nervous system defect. However this usually resolves to its previous state within one or two weeks.

Echocardiography allowed this diagnosis to be made safely and non-invasively with a high degree of reliability. These patients should not be subjected to cardiac catheterisation: left-sided angiography may provoke further peripheral emboli, and opacification of the left side of the heart from a right-sided injection may be associated with spurious filling defects.

COMMENT

As is often the case, the diagnosis of left atrial myxoma is obvious in retrospect. However, the combination of peripheral emboli, changing murmurs and evidence of a systemic disease is very suggestive. Echocardiography allows the diagnosis to be confirmed or excluded with safety.

EXAMINERS' FOLLOW-UP QUESTIONS

1 What other ways can a left atrial myxoma present?
2 What follow-up is required after surgical removal of the tumour?
3 What other types of cardiac tumour can occur?
4 What do you know about mitral leaflet prolapse?
5 How common is central nervous system damage after cardio-pulmonary bypass?

D.G.

Academic decline

WHAT IS THE DIFFERENTIAL DIAGNOSIS?

1   Depressive illness
    Dementia

In a patient of this age with these complaints, the differential diagnosis lies between depressive illness and dementia, the latter term reflecting organic brain disease which may have a wide variety of causes including primary pre-senile dementia (Alzheimer's disease, Pick's disease or Huntington's chorea), alcoholism, hypothyroidism, cerebrovascular disease, cerebral tumour and vitamin deficiencies.

In this patient the associated symptoms of mood disturbance, depressive thinking, and the somatic symptoms of anorexia, weight loss, insomnia and impaired libido strongly suggest a depressive illness, particularly when he reports that these antedate the intellectual complaints.

Patients suffering from dementia often present with symptoms of depression, but in these cases a careful history usually indicates that the intellectual decline had started before the onset of depression. There may be a history of a change in personality, and cognitive impairment is apparent on clinical testing. The patient may be disorientated in time and place, have a poor recall of recent events, and be unable to learn new information accurately.

WHAT ADDITIONAL INVESTIGATIONS WOULD YOU REQUIRE?

1. Interview with patient's spouse
The patient's wife confirmed the gradual onset of depression and social withdrawal 18 months previously, but she maintained that he was considered an effective member of the teaching staff and that there had been no complaints about his academic work. She reported that his physical health has been good and that he drank alcohol very rarely.

2   Mental state assessment
Although the patient expressed a gloomy attitude towards his future he denied suicidal ideation. He was not deluded or hallucinated. Cognitive testing revealed him to be correctly orientated in time and place; he performed accurately but very slowly on the serial sevens test and was able to recall six digits forwards and backwards. He showed a good grasp of current affairs and was able to learn new information accurately. Detailed psychometric assessment was not considered necessary.

3 Family and personal history

It was learned that the patient's father had committed suicide at the age of 60. The patient had been treated by his general practitioner for depression 15 years previously, shortly after he had failed to obtain the post of professor in his department.

4 CT brain scan

This was reported as being completely normal and the result had a reassuring effect on the patient who suspected that he might have developed a cerebral tumour.

WHAT IS THE FINAL DIAGNOSIS?

Depressive illness

HOW WOULD YOU MANAGE THIS PATIENT?

Patients with depressive illness usually respond well to a tricyclic antidepressant. In view of the fact that this patient had a supportive relationship with his wife, and that he had no suicidal thoughts, he was managed as an outpatient. The nature of his illness was discussed with him and he was started on dothiepin 75 mg at night, this being increased to 150 mg at night when the patient was next seen one week later. He was warned about possible anticholinergic side-effects but, apart from a dry mouth and mild blurring of vision, he experienced no problems or untoward effects.

Two weeks after starting treatment he reported that he was less gloomy and that he was sleeping better. After four weeks both he and his wife reported that he was almost back to his usual self, his appetite had improved, he had put on weight, his libido was improving and he could concentrate better. He was able to return to work and he coped effectively with his teaching, research and administrative responsibilities. He continued to worry that he might be forced into early retirement but this did not materialise. Thereafter he was seen each month for supportive psychotherapy and to monitor his progress. He remained well and, after six months, the dose of dothiepin was gradually decreased and tailed off completely over a period of six weeks.

COMMENT

In this patient's case there was evidence that his depression was constitutionally determined in view of his father's suicide but there were also clear triggering factor — namely, failure to achieve academic promotion and the fear of enforced early retirement. In-patient treatment would have been necessary, if the patient had expressed clear suicidal plans or had poor social support. If he had failed to respond to dothiepin, a monoamine oxidase inhibitor or tetracyclic antidepressant could have been tried. Electroconvulsive therapy (ECT) would have been the treatment of choice had he exhibited psychotic features.

EXAMINERS' FOLLOW-UP QUESTIONS

1 What medical conditions make it hazardous to prescribe tricyclic antidepressants?
2 What factors are associated with an increased risk of suicide in patients suffering from depression?
3 What precautions are necessary for patients taking monoamine oxidase inhibitors?
4 With what other somatic symptoms may patients suffering from depression present to a doctor?
5 What are the indications for the prophylactic use of lithium?

G.G.L.

Pyrexia and breathlessness

WHAT IS THE DIFFERENTIAL DIAGNOSIS?

1   Septicaemia
    Acute myocarditis or pericarditis
    Acute infective endocarditis
    Acute rheumatic fever
    Acute aortic valve rupture

In any young patient presenting with cardiovascular collapse, the differential diagnosis lies between hypovolaemia, massive pulmonary embolism, severe ventricular disease, or acute volume overload to the right or left ventricle.

In this patient hypovolaemia is unlikely since the venous pressure was raised, although a minor reduction in plasma volume might have been caused by excessive diuretic therapy. The presence of a normal rather than a reduced pulse volume is very much in favour of acute volume overload to one or other ventricle, rather than intrinsic left or right ventricular disease.

It should be borne in mind that the physical signs of acute valve rupture are frequently quite different from those of the corresponding lesion in its chronic form. In particular, the characteristic murmurs may be absent when valvular regurgitation is total. The associated pyrexia and haematuria obviously makes infective endocarditis much the most likely diagnosis, although it should be noted that acute rheumatic fever may lead to an exactly similar picture.

WHAT ADDITIONAL INVESTIGATIONS WOULD YOU CONSIDER?

1   Chest X-ray
A portable chest X-ray confirmed interstitial pulmonary oedema with lymphatic lines. The heart size was difficult to assess, but was probably a little increased.

2   ECG
The ECG showed sinus tachycardia (115/min). The PR interval was 0.24 sec. There was no evidence of left ventricular hypertrophy, but non-specific T wave changes were present in the lateral chest leads.

3   Urine microscopy
Routine urine testing showed blood + + and protein + . Microscopy revealed red blood cells, but no white cells or casts.

4 Blood cultures

Three sets of blood cultures all showed a heavy growth of *Staphylococcus aureus* sensitive to cloxacillin, flucloxacillin, fusidic acid and gentamicin.

5 Echocardiogram

An urgent M-mode echocardiogram showed disorganisation of the normal aortic valve echogram due to vegetations. The left ventricle was enlarged to 6.3 cm at end-diastole (normal up to 5.5 cm), and the amplitude of wall motion was greatly increased. Premature mitral valve closure was demonstrated, indicating an elevated left ventricular end-diastolic pressure. The presence of aortic valve vegetations was confirmed by two-dimensional echocardiography. In addition, a cavity anterior to the aortic root was demonstrated continuous with the right coronary sinus, suggesting a probable aortic root abscess. Continuous wave Doppler demonstrated equalisation of aortic and ventricular pressures at end-diastole.

6 Plasma digoxin concentration

1.6 ng/ml (therapeutic range 1.0–2.0 ng/ml).

WHAT IS THE FINAL DIAGNOSIS?

Acute staphylococcal endocarditis, causing destruction of the aortic valve and a probable aortic root abscess.

HOW WOULD YOU MANAGE THIS PATIENT?

Traditionally, patients with infective endocarditis were treated for six weeks with intravenous antibiotics, and if evidence of 'heart failure' developed during this period it was managed on conventional lines with digoxin and diuretics. It cannot be stressed too strongly that, in patients with severe valvular regurgitation, this approach to treatment will have a mortality rate approaching 100 per cent. Even if the patient survives the six weeks of antibiotic treatment, the operation is likely to prove fatal due to the irreversible left ventricular damage that had developed during this period.

The case for early operation in this patient is strong, particularly as the echocardiogram shows premature mitral valve closure. Premature aortic valve opening is a similarly bad sign, which implies that the ventricular diastolic pressure is greatly elevated — approaching or equal to that in the aorta so that coronary blood flow will be compromised.

No attempt need be made to control the infection pre-operatively — the only decision is whether to take the patient to theatre on the day of admission, or to wait for 24 hours. A loading dose of an appropriate antibiotic combination should be given with the pre-medication, and at operation the infected valve can be removed, any abscess cavity opened and obliterated, and the valve bed treated with an antiseptic.

Following valve replacement the haemodynamic overload is removed from the left ventricle and a normal circulation is restored. Antibiotic treatment is given for four to six weeks post-operatively. This approach has led to a very substantial increase in survival. In a small minority of patients, post-operative para-prosthetic regurgitation may develop if stitches have to be put into oedematous tissue; this is usually not severe and can be managed medically until it is obliterated at a subsequent operation when the infection has been controlled.

COMMENT

Acute aortic regurgitation may present with an atypical clinical picture, and it should always be suspected when the pulse volume is normal in a patient with cardiovascular collapse. Note that du Rosiez' sign may remain positive: it is a sign of moderately severe aortic regurgitation.

It is clearly important to make an early diagnosis and this is possible using M-mode or two-dimensional echocardiography. As far as possible, invasive investigation should be avoided, due to the risks of either embolism or depression of left ventricular function by the angiographic contrast material.

A long PR interval appearing in a patient with infective endocarditis is ominous, and usually implies an aortic root abscess involving the upper part of the septum and the atrio-ventricular node. Its presence is associated with an increased risk of complete heart block. If it is elected to treat such a patient medically, a temporary pacemaker should be inserted, since a ventricular rate of less than 40/min will prove fatal when there is free aortic regurgitation.

EXAMINERS' FOLLOW-UP QUESTIONS

1   What effect has the introduction of antibiotics had on the pattern of infective endocarditis?
2   How would the clinical picture have differed had the infecting organism been (a) a fungus or (b) a rickettsia?
3   What are the side-effects of the antibiotics that could be used in this patient?
4   What type of acute endocarditis is seen in drug addicts who abuse intravenous drugs?
5   What are the peripheral complications of an acute staphylococcal endocarditis?

D.G.

Cold fingers

WHAT IS THE DIFFERENTIAL DIAGNOSIS?

1   Scleroderma
    Primary Raynaud's disease
    Mixed connective tissue disease

The combination of severe Raynaud's phenomenon with heartburn and dysphagia suggests the diagnosis of scleroderma. Occasionally primary Raynaud's disease can cause severe symptoms and digital ulceration; however this patient's slightly elevated ESR is a clue that there is a systemic illness.

Mixed connective tissue disease is characterised by a clinical overlap between features of scleroderma and systemic lupus erythematosis, and severe Raynaud's phenomenon and synovitis are commonly prominent. In the absence of synovitis or systemic symptoms and signs, this is an unlikely diagnosis.

WHAT ADDITIONAL INVESTIGATIONS WOULD YOU CONSIDER?

1   X-rays of hands
These showed soft tissue swelling around the phalanges with loss of terminal finger pulp. There was resorption of the tufts of the distal phalanges. Periarticular osteoporosis was seen around the interphalangeal joints. No soft tissue clacification was visible.

2   Chest X-ray
The lung fields and heart size were normal. Interstitial fibrosis and secondary pulmonary hypertension are both features of scleroderma, but in this patient there was no evidence of these serious complications.

3   Barium swallow, meal and follow-through
On screening, the oesophageal motility was reduced. On tipping the patient contrast medium was seen to reflux into the oesophagus. The stomach, duodenum and small intestine were all normal, apart from delayed transit of barium through to the terminal ileum. These appearances of decreased peristalsis and intestinal motility are suggestive of scleroderma.

4   Antinuclear antibodies
These were demonstrated by indirect immunofluorescence at a titre of 1:320. Nuclear staining was speckled in pattern. Antinuclear

antibodies may be found in most patients with scleroderma and should not be thought to confirm a diagnosis of either systemic lupus erythematosis or mixed connective tissue disease. The staining pattern is of little clinical significance, all patterns being found in scleroderma and systemic lupus. However, high-titre speckled antinuclear antibodies may suggest the presence of antibodies to ribonucleoprotein (see 5).

5 Antibodies to extractable nuclear antigens

No precipitating antibodies against an extract of calf thymus extract were demonstrated by counterimmuno-electrophoresis. Many independent autoantibodies have been identified in this system. The first to be described was an antibody to a ribonuclease-sensitive antigen (ribonucleoprotein). In high titre, antibodies to ribonuclear protein have a strong association with Raynaud's phenomenon in patients with an overlap condition between systemic lupus and scleroderma: mixed connective tissue disease.

WHAT IS THE FINAL DIAGNOSIS?

Scleroderma, with Raynaud's phenomenon and involvement of the gastrointestinal tract.

HOW WOULD YOU MANAGE THIS PATIENT?

Symptomatic relief is the major aspect of treatment for patients with scleroderma. Avoidance of cold and warm gloves are most important to prevent Raynaud's phenomenon. Treatment for Reynaud's phenomenon are systemically administered prostaglandin or prostacyclin and calcium antagonistics such as nifedipine.

Reflux oesophagitis and dysphagia may be treated with frequent small meals and viscous antacids. Elevation of the bed-head and several pillows may help to prevent noctural reflux. If symptoms are severe, H_2-antagonists such as cimetidine or ranitidine may be of help. A peptic oesophageal stricture can be a serious end-result of uncontrolled gastro-oesophageal reflux. Gut hypomotility is difficult to treat; it has been claimed that metoclopramide is of value, although evidence for this is limited. A low residue diet may help to reduce bloating and constipation.

COMMENT

Although no specific agents presently exist for the treatment of scleroderma, disease progression is slow in most patients. This patient illustrates the typically indolent onset of disease. 10 years later she remained fairly well although she was developing pulmonary fibrosis.

EXAMINERS' FOLLOW-UP QUESTIONS

1   What abnormalities of respiratory function could be found in this patient?
2   Describe the facial signs of scleroderma.
3   Do corticosteroids have a role in the management of scleroderma?
4   Why may a patient with scleroderma develop malabsorption?
5   What form of liver disease is associated with scleroderma?

M.J.W.
G.R.V.H.

Heart failure

WHAT IS THE DIFFERENTIAL DIAGNOSIS?

1   Diffuse impairment of left ventricular function
      Coronary artery disease
    Left ventricular aneurysm
    Acquired ventricular septal defect
    Mitral regurgitation
    Ruptured papillary muscle

The development of cardiac enlargement and pulmonary congestion in a patient following a documented myocardial infarction always requires investigation. The most important differential diagnosis is between diffuse left ventricular disease and one of the surgically correctable complications.

WHAT FURTHER INVESTIGATIONS WOULD YOU CONSIDER?

1   Chest X-ray
The PA chest X-ray showed cardiac enlargement with a cardio-thoracic ratio of 55 per cent (normal < 50 per cent). There was no abnormal prominence on the cardiac border and no intracardiac calcification was seen. The upper lobe vessels were dilated and there were lymphatic lines at the bases, confirming the presence of pulmonary oedema.

2   ECG
The ECG showed QS waves in leads V1–4, with T wave inversion in V5 and V6. There was left atrial hypertrophy.

3   Dynamic cardiac isotope scan
The gated blood pool scan showed left ventricular enlargement with an apical aneurysm. The overall ejection fraction was 35 per cent (normal 55–70 per cent).

4   Two-dimensional echocardiography
This non-invasive procedure confirmed the aneurysm and, in addition, demonstrated a densely-reflecting thrombus at the apex of the ventricle, which was akinetic. The amplitude of the basal wall motion was reduced.

5   Cardiac catheter
At the left heart catheterization, the left ventricular end-diastolic

pressure was 30 mmHg (normal < 12 mmHg). The left ventriculogram confirmed the presence of an apical aneurysm. Function at the base of the heart was felt to be moderately impaired. There was mild mitral regurgitation, but no evidence of a ventricular septal defect. Coronary arteriography showed complete occlusion of the left anterior descending artery just beyond the origin of the first septal branch. The circumflex artery was normal but there was an additional 75 per cent lesion of the right coronary artery.

WHAT IS THE FINAL DIAGNOSIS?

Ventricular aneurysm, due to large anterior myocardial infarction, causing congestive cardiac failure.

HOW WOULD YOU MANAGE THIS PATIENT?

A left ventricular aneurysm may be managed medically or surgically. An operation should be reserved for those patients with dyspnoea or chest pain unresponsive to medical treatment, or for those who have experienced arterial emboli from a ventricular thrombus. Recurrent ventricular arrhythmias usually respond poorly to simple aneurysmectomy.

The presence of additional ventricular disease in this patient (impaired function at the base of the heart) would be a relative contraindication to operation. Medical treatment should be tried first using diuretics and vasodilators, particularly an angiotensin converting enzyme (ACE) inhibitor such as captropril or enalapril given in adequate dosage.

Only if medical treatment fails should surgery be considered. Although the risk of not surviving the operation is small, it provides only symptomatic benefit, and does not improve prognosis. If an aneurysmectomy were performed in this patient, it should be combined with saphenous bypass grafting to the right coronary artery.

A left ventricular aneurysm represents severe ventricular disease. This is reflected in the prognosis, which is poor, with either medical or surgical treatment. A left ventricular aneurysm should be suspected in all patients with coronary artery disease and cardiac enlargement on chest X-ray. It cannot be excluded by the lack of calcification or a discrete bulge on the cardiac contour in the chest X-ray, or by screening the heart; it requires the use of a modern imaging technique such as blood pool scanning, echocardiography, or left ventriculography.

Post-operative studies have shown that ventricular aneurysms frequently recur despite a favourable symptomatic response. Combined medical and surgical treatment may thus be required for optimum management.

EXAMINERS' FOLLOW-UP QUESTIONS

1 What is the characteristic clinical picture of a ruptured papillary muscle?
2 How do the cardiovascular effects of nitrates differ from those of hydralazine or nitroprusside?
3 What is the role of prophylactic beta-adrenergic blockage after myocardial infarction?
4 Discuss the management of recurrent ventricular arrhythmias in such a patient.
5 Should this patient be anticoagulated?

D.G.

Epileptic fit

WHAT IS THE DIFFERENTIAL DIAGNOSIS?

1 Carcinoma of the bronchus
  Pulmonary tuberculosis
2 Inappropriate anti-diuretic hormone secretion

This patient is obviously seriously ill, with an illness that has progressed for some months. The abnormality in the screening tests could be explained by either an oat cell carcinoma of the bronchus or tuberculosis, with associated inappropriate anti-diuretic hormone secretion. The convulsion could be due to either the hyponatraemia, or to cerebral irritation by a tumour or infection.

The patient does not have postural hypotension, hence it is likely that the hyponatraemia is not due to salt deficiency. It is probably due to retention of water.

WHAT ADDITIONAL INVESTIGATIONS WOULD YOU CONSIDER?

1 Chest X-ray
The chest X-ray revealed occlusion of the right main bronchus with collapse of the right lung.

2 Plasma and urine osmolarity
The plasma osmolarity was 242 mosmol/l (normal 285 mosmol/l) and the urinary osmolarity was 580 mosmol/l. Despite the decreased plasma osmolarity, the patient is producing an inappropriately concentrated urine, and thereby retaining water. This abnormality is caused by inappropriate secretion of anti-diuretic hormone.

3 Bronchoscopy
A tumour mass was seen occluding the right main bronchus. A biopsy of the mass revealed spherical, or oat-shaped, cells which were small with deeply-staining nuclei and scanty cytoplasm.

4 CT brain scan
The patient presented with an epileptic fit, but the CT scan showed no abnormality. There was no sign of a cerebral metastasis.

5 EEG
No focal abnormality was detected.

WHAT IS THE FINAL DIAGNOSIS?

Small (oat) cell carcinoma of bronchus, with inappropriate secretion of anti-diuretic hormone, causing a dilutional hyponatraemia and epilepsy.

HOW WOULD YOU MANAGE THIS PATIENT?

This patient's prognosis is poor as oat-cell carcinomas usually arise in the main bronchi and spread rapidly to the regional lymphatics. The pulmonary vessels are involved at an early stage, and widespread haematogenous metastases are frequent.

The inappropriate anti-diuretic hormone secretion (which occurs in one-third of these patients) should gradually respond to water restriction. The patient should be provided with between 500 and 1000 ml of water per day. In addition the patient should receive demethylchlortetracycline (1200 mg per day) which reduces the renal sensitivity to anti-diuretic hormone. Intravenous hypertonic saline should only be given as an emergency measure; this patient presented with epilepsy and should probably receive one litre of 1.8 per cent saline over the 12 hours immediately after admission.

The patient needs effective treatment for the primary tumour. Radiotherapy will reduce the tumour bulk and will allow re-expansion of the collapsed lung. This should be followed by combination chemotherapy usually using four drugs, one of which will be doxorubicin.

The combination of radiotherapy and chemotherapy increases the one-year survival for oat cell carcinoma of the lung from five per cent to 47 per cent.

COMMENT

Abnormal secretion of anti-diuretic hormone or adrenocorticotrophic hormone is usually associated with the small (oat) cell carcinoma of the lung, whereas hypercalcaemia is more common with squamous carcinoma of the lung.

Only 10 per cent of patients with lung cancer survive five years. When first seen only 20 patients in 100 are suitable for surgery, and only six of these are alive at five years. Aggressive combination chemotherapy is a worthwhile beacon of light in this gloomy field of medicine.

EXAMINERS' FOLLOW-UP QUESTIONS

1 Describe the main aetiological factors for carcinoma of the bronchus.

113

2 Does 'passive' cigarette smoking (that is, inhaling other peoples' smoke) increase the chance of lung cancer?

3 What are the main local (intrathoracic) symptoms of carcinoma of the bronchus?

4 What are the main metastatic complications of carcinoma of the bronchus?

5 What are the contraindications to surgery for carcinoma of the bronchus?

D.G.J.

Sudden breathlessness

WHAT IS THE DIFFERENTIAL DIAGNOSIS?

1   Aortic stenosis
     Hypertrophic cardiomyopathy
     Non-rheumatic mitral regurgitation
2   Ischaemic left ventricular disease

Clearly, in view of the combination of the pulse and systolic murmur, the patient has aortic stenosis. However, it is important that hypertrophic cardiomyopathy and non-rheumatic mitral regurgitation are excluded definitively. For the latter to be diagnosed, it is essential that the apical murmur is shown to be pan-systolic. Care should be taken to avoid being misled by the apparent change in quality frequently shown by aortic systolic murmurs when they are conducted to the apex.

The severity of any associated left ventricular disease must also be considered. This is probably significant in this patient as shown by the sustained apex beat, the left atrial impulse, and the accentuated P2. This means that the possibility of associated coronary artery disease must also be considered.

WHAT ADDITIONAL INVESTIGATIONS WOULD YOU CONSIDER?

1   Chest X-ray, PA and lateral
The PA chest X-ray showed a normal heart size and lung fields, but there was definite left atrial enlargement. The lateral chest X-ray showed calcification of the aortic valve.

2   ECG
The ECG showed sinus rhythm, with left atrial hypertrophy. There was poor R-wave progression in leads V2–V4. The QRS voltages were normal, but there was T wave inversion in leads I, aVf, and V4–6.

3   Echocardiogram
This showed a normal left ventricular cavity size. However, there was a significant increase in the thickness of both the septum and posterior left ventricular wall. The mitral valve echo was normal. A two-dimensional echocardiogram confirmed the presence of severe left ventricular hypertrophy. The aortic valve was replaced by a mass of densely reflecting echoes. Continuous wave Doppler cardiogram demonstrated greatly increased blood velocity across the aortic valve — 5 m.sec^{-1} corresponding to a pressure gradient of 100 mmHg.

4 Cardiac catheterisation

The right heart pressures were normal. The left ventricular pressures were 220/5, with an end-diastolic pressure of 15 mmHg. As the aortic pressure was 120/80 there was a considerable pressure gradient (100 mmHg) across the aortic value due to the severe stenosis. The left ventriculogram showed a small left ventricular cavity due to ventricular hypertrophy with enlarged papillary muscles. The aortogram showed trivial aortic regurgitation, and the coronary arteriograms were normal.

WHAT IS THE FINAL DIAGNOSIS?

Severe aortic stenosis with left ventricular hypertrophy.

HOW WOULD YOU MANAGE THIS PATIENT?

This patient requires early aortic valve replacement since he is at risk from sudden death, or at least further attacks of acute pulmonary oedema (which was the basis of his presenting symptom). Even in the absence of symptoms, patients with significant aortic stenosis should be considered for operation, since progressive deterioration of left ventricular function is likely to occur over a period of six to 12 months.

COMMENT

This patient presents with a classical history of aortic stenosis. Alternative presentations include typical angina pectoris or syncope, particularly associated with unaccustomed exertion. Unfortunately there is good evidence to suggest that large numbers of such patients are still present, undetected, in the adult population of the United Kingdom.

EXAMINERS' FOLLOW-UP QUESTIONS

1   What is the aetiology of calcific aortic stenosis?
2   What advice do you give a patient with a prosthetic aortic valve?
3   How would the clinical picture have differed if the patient had had fixed sub-aortic stenosis?
4   Do patients with aortic stenosis, who develop anginal pain, always have coronary disease?
5   What is the significance of an 'a' wave in the jugular venous pulse of a patient with left ventricular hypertrophy?

D.G.

Jaundice in a sauna secretary

WHAT IS THE DIFFERENTIAL DIAGNOSIS?

1 Acute alcoholic hepatitis
   Virus hepatitis

The combination of a history of alcohol excess with dependence (morning drinking, tremor with abstinence), jaundice, florid vascular spiders, tender hepatomegaly, macrocytosis, fever and leukocytosis strongly suggests the diagnosis of acute alcoholic hepatitis.

Virus hepatitis is unlikely in view of the florid vascular spiders, the very large liver, the relatively low aspartate transaminase, the leukocytosis and the macrocytosis.

WHAT ADDITIONAL INVESTIGATIONS WOULD YOU CONSIDER?

1 Prothrombin time and platelet count
The prothrombin time was 24 seconds with a control of 13 seconds; it failed to correct with 10 mg vitamin K intramuscularly for three days. The platelet count was $310 \times 10^9/l$.

2 Hepatitis B surface antigen
Alcoholic and viral liver disease may coexist. This patient worked in an environment where hepatitis B carriage is frequent (sauna, homosexuals etc). In fact the radioimmunoassay for hepatitis B surface antigen was negative.

3 EEG
This showed a slowing of the mean frequency to 6 cycles/second (normal 8–13 cycles/second), indicating mild hepatic encephalopathy. Care would be needed with her dietary protein intake.

4 Liver scan
This showed virtually no hepatic uptake of isotope and was compatible with severe hepatocellular disease, such as acute alcoholic hepatitis. A liver scan may be useful as an indicator of hepatocellular disease when liver biopsy is impossible, as in this patient, because of impaired blood coagulation.

5 Upper gastrointestinal endoscopy
No oesophageal varices were seen. This is in accord with the absence of splenomegaly.

6 Serum B12 and folate levels

Surprisingly, these were normal. Folate deficiency is common in alcoholics, and the serum B12 is often elevated with hepatocellular damage.

7 Blood cultures

This patient was pyrexial, and septicaemia is frequent in any patient with advanced hepatocellular disease. The blood cultures were negative. 'Spontaneous' bacterial peritonitis should also be considered. However, the ascites was minimal and a diagnostic tap was not considered necessary. The pyrexia was presumably due to hepatocellular necrosis.

8 CT scan of the abdomen

This is not essential, but if available can be used to measure liver fat content. In this patient, the liver attenutation value was 8–10 EV (normal 28–33 EV). This indicates gross fatty infiltration of the liver. The liver was smooth and enlarged. The spleen was not enlarged. After intravenous contrast, the portal vein was seen to be patent and no portal-systemic collaterals could be seen.

9 Serum cholesterol

This was normal. Increased concentrations are found in alcoholics with Zieve's syndrome, where haemolysis may occur and pancreatic damage is usually present.

10 Liver biopsy

A coincidental cirrhosis cannot be excluded at this stage without a liver biopsy. This was impossible to perform at the time of this patient's admission. In any case it would not affect the immediate management. If considered essential for accurate diagnosis, it could have been performed by the transjugular route.

WHAT IS THE FINAL DIAGNOSIS?

Acute alcoholic hepatitis.

HOW WOULD YOU MANAGE THIS PATIENT?

The patient must abstain immediately and totally from alcohol. A watch must be kept for the development of withdrawal symptoms (anxiety, tachycardia, tremor). The prophylactic use of chlormethiazole must be considered. However, the use of this drug, or an alternative such as diazepam, may precipitate hepatic encephalopathy. In fact this patient did not develop the symptoms of alcohol withdrawal (delirium tremens).

Complete bed rest should be enforced. High-dose polyvitamins should be given intravenously for seven days, and followed by a potent oral vitamin B preparation. Oral folic acid supplements should also be given.

This patient is anorexic and continuously nauseated. She should be fed for 10 days via a thin nasogastric tube, with a diet containing 2000 calories and 60 g protein daily. Dietary salt should be restricted to 22.5 mmol daily and fluid intake to one litre daily. Potassium chloride supplements (100 mmol daily) should be given for the first five days. Intravenous branched-chain amino acids are not necessary.

In view of the severe malnutrition it was decided to give a relatively high protein intake, despite the mild hepatic encephalopathy. In the event the encephalopathy did not progress. She improved slowly so that over the next five weeks the pyrexia and nausea subsided, the serum bilirubin had fallen to 52 μmol/l, and the prothrombin time was reduced to three seconds over control. At this time a liver biopsy could be performed, which showed severe hepatitis of the alcoholic type with much fatty change; fibrosis was extensive in Zone III (centrizonal) but cirrhosis was not clearly evident. There was moderate siderosis. After eight weeks she was discharged from hospital, much improved.

COMMENT

This young woman suffered from a remarkably severe acute alcoholic hepatitis. It followed 13 years of social drinking and five years of heavy intake. Women may be more susceptible to alcoholic liver damage than men.

The liver lesion had not yet reached the stage of cirrhosis and, with total abstinence from alcohol, complete reversion to normal is possible.

Three months later she was abstinent and back to full-time work. The total bilirubin was 21 μmol/l. However, six months after discharge from hospital, she started drinking alcohol again at weekends. Her aspartate transaminase was 26 U/l, the γ glutamyl transpeptidase 274 U/l (normal 10–48 U/l), and the MCV 106 fl. The prognosis must be guarded.

EXAMINERS' FOLLOW-UP QUESTIONS

1 Outline possible measures to prevent this patient returning to alcohol abuse.
2 Why was her blood macrocytic?
3 Why was she hypokalaemic?
4 What is the place of intravenous amino acids in treating such a patient?
5 Discuss the use of serum γ glutamyl transpeptidase as a screening test for alcoholism.

S.S.

Nausea and vomiting

WHAT IS THE DIFFERENTIAL DIAGNOSIS?

1 Hypercalcaemia
   Hyperparathyroidism
   Malignancy
     Myelomatosis
     Bony metastases
   Vitamin D intoxication
   Sarcoidosis
   Thyrotoxicosis

The differential diagnosis of isolated nausea and vomiting, without any additional symptoms, includes uraemia, hypercalcaemia, raised intracranial pressure, alcoholism and stress. The screening test results provide the major clue for this patient's initial diagnosis. Indeed, without the screening tests it would be impossible to make any definite diagnosis.

The combination of marked hypercalcaemia, a low phosphate and an elevated chloride, make hyperparathyroidism the most likely diagnosis. In view of this patient's age, malignancy must be the other possible cause of hypercalcaemia. However, the screening test results are otherwise normal. The patient has a high haemoglobin due to dehydration, a normal ESR, a normal total protein, and a normal alkaline phosphatase.

The most common presentation of primary hyperparathyroidism is asymptomatic hypercalcaemia found on a routine biochemistry screen. Renal calculi, bone disease, gastrointestinal disturbance and psychiatric problems are much rarer modes of presentation.

A careful history should be taken to exclude overdosing with 'health food' vitamin supplements: vitamin D intoxication can cause profound and sustained hypercalcaemia.

WHAT ADDITIONAL INVESTIGATIONS WOULD YOU CONSIDER?

1 Repeat biochemistry screen after rehydration
It is sensible to exclude changes merely due to dehydration. After an intravenous infusion of 3 litres of 0.9% sodium chloride, the urea dropped to 7.4 mmol/l, but the calcium remained elevated at 3.63 mmol/l.

2 Parathyroid hormone (PTH)
The plasma concentration of parathyroid hormone can be measured by radioimmunoassay. This patient's PTH concentration was

80 pg/ml, (upper limit of normal, 85 pg/ml), which is towards the upper limit of normal and inappropriate for the high plasma calcium. This concentration of parathyroid hormone suggests the diagnosis of primary hyperparathyroidism.

Hypercalcaemia due to malignancy is usually associated with a marked suppression of plasma parathyroid hormone concentration.

3 Selective neck vein catheterisation

Catheterisation of the veins of the thyroid, with multiple blood samples for parathyroid hormone assay, may provide localisation of a para-thyroid adenoma. The highest concentrations of the parathyroid hormone were found draining the right upper quadrant of the thyroid bed.

4 Ultrasound examination of the neck

A skilful ultrasonographer can sometimes detect a parathyroid adenoma, providing additional pre-operative information to the surgeon. Examination of this patient's neck suggested that the right upper parathyroid gland was enlarged.

WHAT IS THE FINAL DIAGNOSIS?

Hypercalcaemia due to primary hyperparathyroidism, secondary to a right superior parathyroid adenoma.

HOW WOULD YOU MANAGE THIS PATIENT?

The patient needs urgent rehydration with 0.9% sodium chloride, taking care not to overload her circulation in view of her age. When she has been fully rehydrated, a small oral dose of frusemide may be given to initiate a diuresis. Obviously this diuresis must be compensated by additional intravenous fluids.

The more aggressive management of severe hypercalcaemia using calcitonin and mithramycin would probably not be needed for this patient. These agents are often necessary for hypercalcaemia due to malignancy.

There is no medical treatment for hyperparathyroidism. This patient is symptomatic, and she needs surgical exploration of her neck to remove the parathyroid adenoma. There is a 90 per cent chance it will be a single parathyroid adenoma; three per cent of the tumours may be multiple and only two per cent are malignant. About five per cent of patients have hyperplasia of all four glands.

COMMENT

The management of the patient with asymptomatic primary hyper-parathyroidism remains uncertain. A conservative opinion would recommend regular review of the serum calcium and renal function, but an alternative approach would be early surgical exploration of the neck. The major difficulty is that a mild degree of hyperparathyroidism is relatively common. A simple guideline for choosing a surgical approach is a plasma calcium concentration of greater than 3.0 mmol/l and a significantly diminished bone density.

Hyperparathyroidism may occasionally be associated with either thyrotoxicosis or multiple endocrine adenomatosis. If a patient with hypercalcaemia also has a peptic ulcer, the fasting plasma gastrin should be measured. Conversely, patients with peptic ulcer should have their plasma calcium measured.

It is worth noting that 24 hour urinary calcium excretion and steroid suppression tests are no longer used as investigations of hypercalcaemia. The former is not dependable and the latter unnecessary.

EXAMINERS' FOLLOW-UP QUESTIONS

1 How would you manage tetany in this patient's early postoperative period?
2 Why does hypercalcaemia damage the kidneys?
3 What do you know about the metabolism of vitamin D?
4 What is meant by the terms 'secondary' and 'tertiary' hyperparathyroidism?
5 Why may patients with malignancy have a high plasma calcium?

P.D.

The dangers of exercise

WHAT IS THE DIFFERENTIAL DIAGNOSIS?

1   Hypertrophic cardiomyopathy
    Aortic stenosis
    Coronary artery disease
    Mitral regurgitation

The combination of chest pain and exercise-induced syncope in a young patient with a family history of sudden death, along with left ventricular hypertrophy and a systolic murmur, all suggest hypertrophic cardiomyopathy. The history of rheumatic fever is probably irrelevant, and is frequently obtained from patients with systolic murmurs arising from a variety of causes. The normal pulse excludes aortic stenosis.

WHAT ADDITIONAL INVESTIGATIONS WOULD YOU CONSIDER?

1   Chest X-ray
The heart size was normal, and the lung fields clear.

2   ECG
The ECG showed left axis deviation (– 40 degrees), but was otherwise normal.

3   Echocardiogram
This showed severe left ventricular hypertrophy involving both the septum and the posterior wall. In addition, there was systolic anterior movement of the anterior cusp of the mitral valve. The aortic valve showed mid-systolic closure. Two-dimensional echocardiography demonstrated generalised involvement of the left ventricle, with apical cavity obliteration at end-systole. Continuous Doppler wave demonstrated a left ventricular outflow gradient of 60 mmHg.

4   A 24-hour tape
Frequent ventricular ectopic beats, a short episode of atrial fibrillation, and several salvoes of ventricular tachycardia, lasting up to six beats, were recorded during the 24 hours.

5   Exercise test
A standardised Bruce protocol exercise test showed the patient able to complete Stage IV (normal). However, runs of ectopic beats and several episodes of ventricular tachycardia occurred during recovery.

123

WHAT IS THE FINAL DIAGNOSIS?

Hypertrophic cardiomyopathy, with left ventricular outflow tract obstruction and ventricular arrhythmias.

HOW WOULD YOU MANAGE THIS PATIENT?

Further diagnostic manoeuvres, such as cardiac catheterisation or endomyocardial biopsy, are probably not indicated except as research procedures.

Chest pain in hypertrophic cardiomyopathy may respond to beta-blockers. In addition there is evidence to suggest that these drugs may modify favourably the diastolic properties of the left ventricle, which are a major cause of symptoms in this condition. More recently, similar beneficial effects from calcium-blocking drugs have been reported. Ventricular arrhythmias and, in particular, overall prognosis are not improved by the routine administration of beta-blocking drugs. However, for this patient in whom arrhythmias seem to have been provoked by exertion, it might be worth repeating the exercise test after beta blockade.

Recent evidence suggests that amiodarone, at a dose of 600 mg/day, may reduce the frequency of ventricular arrhythmias recorded during 24-hour monitoring. Whether amiodarone improves prognosis remains to be seen. Surgical resection of the hypertrophic septal myocardium, to reduce the outflow tract gradient, probably has little to offer these patients.

COMMENT

This patient represents a very characteristic clinical presentation of hypertrophic cardiomyopathy. The focus of interest in such cases has shifted away from the outflow tract gradient as a source of morbidity, and is now concentrated on the abnormal diastolic properties of the ventricle, and the increased incidence of severe ventricular arrhythmias. Angina is common and, as in aortic stenosis, this can coexist with a normal coronary arteriogram.

EXAMINERS' FOLLOW-UP QUESTIONS

1   The patient had read that long-distance running prevents the development of coronary artery disease. Would you agree with this idea? What advice would you give him about exercise in the future?
2   What is the inheritance of hypertrophic cardiomyopathy?
3   What may the ECG show in hypertrophic cardiomyopathy?
4   Why might the calcium-blocking drugs be of value in the treatment of hypertrophic cardiomyopathy?
5   What is this patient's prognosis?

D.G.

Loss of weight and height

WHAT IS THE DIFFERENTIAL DIAGNOSIS?

1. Carcinoma of the bronchus
   Carcinoma of the prostate
   Myelomatosis

Recurrent bronchitis in a man of this age suggests a bronchial carcinoma. Prostatic symptoms, albuminuria and recurrent urinary tract infections point to a possible prostatic carcinoma, although he is a little young. The high ESR, anaemia and backache could suggest vertebral metastases from either type of carcinoma but, if this were so, one would expect a raised alkaline phosphatase to go with the hypercalcaemia of malignancy. The patient has a high total protein (95 g/l): myelomatosis must be excluded.

WHAT ADDITIONAL INVESTIGATIONS WOULD YOU CONSIDER?

1 Chest X-ray
Despite the repeated chest infections, the chest X-ray was normal.

2 Serum acid phosphatase
This was normal, however this does not completely exclude involvement of the spine by metastases from prostatic carcinoma.

3 X-ray of the spine
There were several scattered osteolytic lesions, which the radiologist reported as consistent with metastases or myelomatosis.

4 Bone marrow
The bone marrow was heavily infiltrated with plasma cells, many of which had abnormal morphology. Some centres are able to perform immunofluorescence with specific antisera, demonstrating in myelomatosis that the great majority of the plasma cells contain only one class of immunoglobulin. This patient's plasma cells contained IgG.

5 Serum protein electrophoresis
A monoclonal band was demonstrated.

6 Serum immunoglobulins

IgA: 0.5 g/l (normal: 0.5–4.0 g/l)

IgG: 38 g/l (normal: 5.0–15 g/l)

IgM: 0.4 g/l (normal: 0.6–2.8 g/l)

The IgG is elevated; the patient has a monoclonal band: he has IgG myelomatosis.

7 Urine for Bence Jones protein

The patient's urine contained Bence Jones protein — now known to be free light chains. Immunological studies showed that they were *kappa* chains.

WHAT IS THE FINAL DIAGNOSIS

Myelomatosis (IgG with *kappa* chain Bence Jones protein), with associated bone metastases, anaemia, hypercalcaemia and renal failure.

HOW WOULD YOU MANAGE THIS PATIENT?

The long-term aim of treatment is to reduce the total mass of tumour in the body, which may allow reversal of some of the side-effects caused by its presence. Continuous low-dose cyclophosphamide or melphalan may be used, or monthly intravenous treatment with vincristine and Adriamycin, and oral dexamethasone (VAD regimen).

This patient's bone pain may either be helped by indomethacin, or perhaps radiotherapy to a localised area of particular discomfort.

The patient is anaemic and needs a blood transfusion. He may need repeated transfusions until the chemotherapy has reduced the size of the tumour mass in the bone marrow, which is squeezing out the normal marrow.

The hypercalcaemia should also improve as the tumour mass recedes, but the patient should maintain a good diuresis by taking a high fluid intake. This may also reduce renal damage caused by the Bence Jones light chains.

The patient presented with recurrent chest infections, but unfortunately prophylaxis with gammaglobulin injections is not very effective. The patient will need vigorous treatment with antibiotics whenever he develops a chest infection. Intravenous fresh frozen plasma should be given if he develops pneumonia.

COMMENT

Surprisingly, in myelomatosis the presence of bone lesions or hypercalcaemia, or the serum concentration of the paraprotein, do not correlate with survival. However, prognosis in myeloma is bad if one or more of the following is present at the time of diagnosis: a low serum albumin, an elevated plasma urea, Bence Jones protein in the urine, or anaemia (less than 7.5 g/dl). It is clear that this patient has a poor prognosis.

Treatment should be monitored by serial measurement of the abnormal paraprotein, which should drop by about 50 per cent in the first three months of treatment. In addition, the haemoglobin, urea and calcium should be measured regularly.

The average patient with myeloma survives about three years. Death is usually due to increasing tumour mass, or the tumour becoming more aggressive, or renal failure due to Bence Jones proteinuria, infection or amyloid kidney.

Myelomatosis may be difficult to distinguish from carcinomatosis, before the results of bone marrow or protein electrophoresis are available. Two important clues may come from the screening tests: in myelomatosis the ESR is usually much elevated but the alkaline phosphatase is usually normal; in carcinomatosis the alkaline phosphatase is usually elevated, with only a moderate change of ESR.

EXAMINERS' FOLLOW-UP QUESTIONS

1   What would you do if this patient's calcium was 3.80 mmol/l?
2   What are the symptoms of blood hyperviscosity due to IgG myelomatosis?
3   Why did this patient present with a plasma sodium of 127 mmol/l?
4   What would you do if this patient suddenly developed a spastic paraplegia?
5   How would you manage a *Herpes zoster* infection in an immunocompromised patient?

D.G.J.

A lump in the neck

WHAT IS THE DIFFERENTIAL DIAGNOSIS?

1 Lymphoma
   Hodgkin's disease
   Non-Hodgkin's lymphoma
2 Lymphadenopathy due to infection
   Infectious mononucleosis
   Cytomegalovirus
   Toxoplasmosis
   Tuberculosis
   Acquired immune deficiency syndrome (AIDS)

A combination of alcohol-related chest pain and cervical lymph node enlargement strongly suggests Hodgkin's disease. With the splenic enlargement, and the history of fever and night sweats, this is clinically stage IIIB, although there has been no weight loss. Alcohol-induced pain is occasionally reported in non-Hodgkin's lymphomas and in sarcoidosis.

Tender lymph nodes are more likely to be associated with an infection, but examination of his mouth and pharynx did not reveal tonsillar enlargement or the presence of an exudate; no rash was noted. He did not keep domestic animals at home, which might have been important if toxoplasmosis was being considered. The history is rather short for tuberculosis. AIDS must be a possible diagnosis.

WHAT FURTHER INVESTIGATIONS WOULD YOU CONSIDER?

1 Chest X-ray
'A left hilar mass is present. A lymphoma must be excluded. Tomograms are indicated.'

Tomograms were done and the radiologist's opinion was that the possible increase in soft tissue shadowing at the site was due to the left pulmonary artery passing over the left main stem bronchus. The 'mass' did not have the clearly convex margin characteristic of lymph-adenopathy. 40–50 per cent of patients with Hodgkin's disease do have mediastinal adenopathy demonstrated on the chest radiograph at the time of presentation.

2 Blood film
Atypical lymphoid cells were not seen: infectious mononucleosis, cyto-megalovirus and toxoplasmosis can be eliminated.

3 Antibody to human immune deficiency virus (HIV)

An urgent result reported that the antibody was not present. This does not eliminate early infection with HIV, but it eliminates AIDS as the cause of this illness.

4 Biopsy of right supraclavicular node

'There is loss of normal lymph node architecture, due to nodular-sclerosing Hodgkin's disease, with the nodules showing the features of a mixed cellularity type.'

In nodular-sclerosing Hodgkin's disease the dominant feature is dense bands of collagen traversing the lymph node, which isolate the abnormal lymphoid tissue. The cell pattern within these nodules may take the form of lymphocyte predominant, mixed cellularity, or lymphocyte depletion. This sub-classification has some prognostic significance, with a progressively poorer outlook for those patients with fewer lymphocytes in the nodes.

5 Bone marrow aspiration and trephine biopsy

The aspirate showed the reactive features of 'chronic disease', with iron being present only in the macrophages. The histology of the trephine biopsy taken from the iliac crest did not show involvement by Hodgkin's disease. A positive trephine biopsy is found in fewer than 5 per cent of patients with Hodgkin's disease, whereas there is involvement of the bone marrow in at least 40 per cent of non-Hodgkin's lymphomas at presentation.

6 Lymphogram

There was good filling of nodes to the level of L2; the para aortic nodes were normal but there was a node in the left iliac chain whose appearance was equivocal. The features of disease affecting lymph nodes is firstly an increase in size and roundness of the node, which loses its usual oblong shape; secondly, an abnormal pattern becomes apparent. A plain film should be repeated in two, four and eight weeks' time, so that any abnormality can be confirmed; lymph node patterns are never static.

7 Intravenous urography

There was no evidence of hydronephrosis, nor displacement or obstruction of the ureters. An IVU is complementary to the lymphogram.

8 Abdominal ultrasound

No abnormality was demonstrated in the liver, spleen or para-aortic region. Lesions in the liver and spleen are usually too small or diffuse to be demonstrated, but enlarged lymph nodes can be visualised if they are at least 2 cm in diameter.

9 CT scan

Where this investigation is available, it offers more precision than ultrasound, but it should not displace ultrasound examination. It is particularly valuable when intrathoracic, intraabdominal or hepatic disease is present.

10   Staging laparotomy

No macroscopic abnormality was noted in the gastrointestinal tract; the liver and pancreas appeared normal, the lymph nodes were normal in size, but the spleen appeared slightly enlarged. The spleen was removed; a clip was placed on the splenic pedicle. The spleen weighed 203 g (normal 100–250 g). A wedge and a needle biopsy of the liver was taken; lymph nodes from the upper and lower paraaortic groups and from the mesentery were excised. The histology of all these tissues showed them to be free from involvement by Hodgkin's disease.

The clinical staging, which was determined by the finding of disease on both sides of the diaphragm (involved cervical lymph nodes and apparent splenomegaly), was stage III. This was not changed by the findings in the laboratory tests, the bone marrow biopsy, or by the lymphogram and X-ray studies. The final staging is wholly determined by the results of the staging laparotomy and the pathological assessment of the tissues removed. Ultimately, it is the pathological stage which will determine therapy.

WHAT IS THE FINAL DIAGNOSIS?

Hodgkin's disease, stage IIB.

HOW WOULD YOU MANAGE THIS PATIENT?

With the revision of the staging, following the pathological assessment of the resected tissues, there was a clear case for radiotherapy. He received mantle irradiation. He tolerated this well but within three months, he complained again of alcohol-induced pain, localised to the abdomen and mid-back, for which he required analgesics. When examined, lymph nodes were present in the left axilla and in the groin. Unfortunately, a repeat plain X-ray of his abdomen showed that very little contrast medium remained in the nodes. An abdominal ultrasound revealed nodal enlargement, a finding which was confirmed by repeating the lymphogram. Soon, evidence of further node enlargement was found in other areas, on both sides of the diaphragm. Treatment with multiple cytotoxic agents was started.

COMMENT

Hodgkin's disease is potentially curable where the disease is limited, and, in general, the results of staging correlate with the prognosis. Whatever the impression gained by clinical examination, pathological staging remains the criterion which determines the type of treatment the patient should receive.

Positive laparotomy findings are found in about one half of stage IIB patients. In stage III (A and B), positive splenic histology is found in about 75% of A and 90% of B patients respectively.

Did intraabdominal disease exist in this patient at the time of laparotomy? In spite of examining many thin slices of the spleen, it is quite possible that a focus of Hodgkin's disease was missed. Likewise, it is probable that in many hospitals only one or two sections of a lymph node are looked at. Ten percent of patients with para aortic node involvement do not have splenic disease. Also, in about a third of patients, assessment of intraabdominal disease is wrong.

The role of a staging laparotomy is controversial, and is being reconsidered. If therapy will be affected by the results, then clearly an indication exists. The need is unlikely in patients with stage IIIB or IV, for the elderly, and probably for most children. This patient had splenomegaly, and clinical considerations on the extent of the disease created an element of doubt.

Results from the Royal Marsden Hospital show that about 70 per cent of patients with stage I and II disease remain disease-free after radiotherapy. Radiotherapy is often supplemented with six courses of combination chemotherapy and, although it is early to assess, it appears that survival is improved significantly. Stage IV patients usually receive only combination chemotherapy.

EXAMINERS' FOLLOW-UP QUESTIONS

1 Is there any relationship between tonsillectomy and the development of Hodgkin's disease?
2 What are the rules about counselling before a blood test for AIDS (anti-HIV)?
3 What are the differences between Stages I to IV, A and B?
4 What is the 'classical' pattern of fever associated with Hodgkin's disease?
5 What are the complications of a splenectomy?

E.J.P.-W.

Over-activity following childbirth

WHAT IS THE DIFFERENTIAL DIAGNOSIS?

1 Manic illness
Schizophrenia
Toxic confusional state

The most likely diagnosis in this case was a manic illness developing shortly after childbirth. Schizophrenia has to be considered in view of the grandiose delusions but there were no other characteristic features such as thought disorder, passivity of feelings or auditory hallucinations. She did not show any evidence of impaired consciousness, disturbance of memory of perceptual abnormalities to support a diagnosis of an acute confusional state.

WHAT ADDITIONAL INVESTIGATIONS WOULD YOU REQUIRE?

1 Family history of psychiatric illness
There was a strong family history in that her mother and older brother had both received treatment for depression, and there was a suggestion that her brother had also experienced brief episodes of hypomania although he had not come to medical attention for these.

2 Previous history and pre-morbid personality
Further information indicated that the patient had suffered two episodes of depression at the ages of 21 and 23, there being no obvious precipitating factor on either occasion. She required hospital admission for each episode and on the second occasion was treated with electroconvulsive therapy (ECT). Apart from these illnesses she appeared to have a stable personality and to have had a successful career at school and teacher training college. There had been no marital problems and the pregnancy had been planned. She did not abuse alcohol or other drugs.

WHAT IS THE FINAL DIAGNOSIS?

Manic illness occurring in puerperium.

HOW WOULD YOU MANAGE THIS PATIENT?

The severity of the patient's illness required that she be admitted to hospital. After persuasion from her husband and relatives she agreed to admission to the psychiatric unit. No mother and baby facilities were available but her husband arranged to take time off work to look after the baby at home. The patient was treated with chlorpromazine in doses up to 600 mg daily. Daily contact with her baby was maintained and within a week her mental state had improved sufficiently for her to be able to take an increasingly active part in her baby's care under nursing supervision. The dose of chlorpromazine was gradually reduced and tailed off completely.

Before her discharge home the nature of her illness and the likelihood of recurrent episodes were discussed with the patient and her husband and it was agreed that she be treated with prophylactic lithium carbonate.

COMMENT

This patient experienced the severest form of psychiatric illness following childbirth, namely postpartum psychosis. This can take the form of an affective illness (as in this case with hypomanic symptoms), schizophrenia or rarely an acute confusional state. Approximately two women in every thousand require admission to a psychiatric hospital for a psychotic illness which develops within the first few weeks of the puerperium. The immediate prognosis is usually good but there is a twenty per cent risk of recurrence after further deliveries. The decision to treat this patient prophylactically with lithium was based on the previous personal history and family history of affective illness.

EXAMINERS' FOLLOW-UP QUESTIONS

1 What are the other psychological complications of childbirth?
2 What are the complications of treatment with chlorpromazine?
3 What precautions have to be taken before starting a patient on lithium?
4 What are the long-term complications of lithium therapy?
5 What advice would you give this patient if she wishes to have further children?

G.G.L.

A multisystem disease?

WHAT IS THE DIFFERENTIAL DIAGNOSIS?

1 The nephritic syndrome
   Acute post-streptococcal glomerulonephritis
   Interstitial nephritis (post-streptococcal or penicillin-induced polyarteritis)
   Systemic lupus erythematosus
   Henoch–Schönlein purpura
   Wegener's granulomatosis
   Subacute bacterial endocarditis
2 Accelerated phase hypertension

Oliguria with haematuria, proteinuria and moderate oedema, together with hypertension and impaired renal function, constitute the nephritic syndrome. This has developed in a young man some 10 days after an upper respiratory tract infection, which must make a post-streptococcal glomerulonephritis the most likely diagnosis. Rashes are not uncommon with many acute streptococcal infections and therefore it does not necessarily mean that in this patient there is a complicating allergic reaction to penicillin. Although a course of penicillin will eradicate the streptococcal infection it has no influence on the incidence or severity of any subsequent glomerulonephritis. It may however make it more difficult to diagnose, as the antibiotic therapy will lower the antibody titres associated with the streptococcal infection.

An allergic interstitial nephritis may occur after a streptococcal infection or penicillin therapy. Eosinophilia and eosinophiluria may point to this diagnosis. A salt-losing polyuric state usually develops with plasma volume depletion, rather than the volume expansion seen in this patient. A renal biopsy is needed to diagnose an interstitial nephritis.

Joint pains, rashes and a nephritic illness may be produced by several multisystem diseases, for example, polyarteritis, Henoch–Schönlein purpura, systemic lupus erythematosus or Wegener's granulomatosis. Polyarteritis is usually associated with a neutrophilia. It is unusual for Henoch–Schönlein purpura to present with severe renal impairment but it may occur, particularly in older patients. The rash is usually characteristic, with palpable purpuric spots over the lower legs, ankles and buttocks. Systemic lupus erythematosus is unusual in males, but may occur. This patient's mild upper respiratory tract symptoms are insufficient to warrant a diagnosis of Wegener's granulomatosis. It is common to find abnormal liver function tests (raised alkaline phosphatase) in Wegener's granulomatosis. Occasional patients with subacute bacterial endocarditis have prominent extra-cardiac features which will include glomerulonephritis. The absence of either fever or a heart murmur makes bacterial endocarditis extremely unlikely.

WHAT ADDITIONAL INVESTIGATIONS WOULD YOU CONSIDER?

1 Urine microscopy
10 ml of fresh urine should be centrifuged at 1000 rpm for five minutes. The sediment should be gently resuspended in 0.5 ml of urine and one drop placed on a microscope slide and examined carefully under the high power of the microscope. This patient's urine contained red cells, tubular cells, hyaline and granular casts. Numerous red cell casts were also seen. It is now usual to examine the urine deposit under phase contrast. This may reveal dysmorphic red cells, whose membrane is damaged and shape distorted by passage through an inflamed glomerulus. These last findings mean glomerular bleeding and is almost diagnostic of glomerulonephritis.

2 24-hour urine collection
A 24-hour urine collection should be sent for creatinine clearance and total protein. This patient's renal function was severely impaired with a creatinine clearance of 23 ml/min (normal > 90 ml/min); he was losing 3 g protein per 24 hours.

3 Anti-streptolysin 'O' titre
It is unlikely that the titre would be high in a patient who has received a prompt course of penicillin. Nevertheless if paired sera are taken, on admission and 10 days later, a significant change is strong confirmatory evidence for the diagnosis of a recent streptococcal infection.

4 Throat swab
At this stage, after penicillin therapy, the throat swab was negative. Culture of a group A, beta-haemolytic *Streptococci* would of course support the diagnosis.

5 Immunological studies
Circulating immune complexes may be detected by a variety of tests. These tests are not widely available as none is really satisfactory for day-to-day clinical use. Indirect evidence of the formation of immune complexes can be gained from the finding of a positive rheumatoid factor, from the presence of cryoglobulins in the plasma, and also a low C3. In this patient cryoglobulins were present and the plasma C3 was markedly depressed. The sheep cell agglutination test for rheumatoid factor was positive at a titre of 128, but autoantibodies (antinuclear factor, etc) were negative. The finding of a low C3 in nephritis is helpful as it occurs in the following conditions:
  i   Acute post-infectious glomerulonephritis
 ii   Mesangiocapillary glomerulonephritis

iii Subacute bacterial endocarditis and shunt nephritis
iv Cryoglobulinaemia
v Systemic lupus erythematosus

6 Renal biopsy

In a clear-cut case of classical acute post-streptococcal glomerulonephritis a renal biopsy is not necessary, unless renal function is
seriously deranged or recovery unduly slow. In this case a renal
biopsy was done as the ASO titre and throat swab were negative. For
maximum information and to ensure a diagnosis, renal biopsy tissue
must be processed for light, electron and immunofluorescent
microscopy.

This biopsy showed a diffuse endocapillary proliferative
glomerulonephritis, with numerous polymorphonuclear leucocytes in
the capillary loops (exudative). Electron microscopy showed large
electron-dense deposits along the glomerular basement membrane
beneath the epithelial cells. Immunofluorescence was strongly
positive with IgG and C3 deposited in coarse blobs around the
capillary loops. This discontinuous or granular distribution of immune
reactants is typical of an immune complex type of reaction. This is in
sharp contrast to the linear immunofluorescence, when biopsy
material is stained for IgG, in Goodpasture's syndrome where there is
an antibody directed against the glomerular basement membrane.
This patient's biopsy had the typical features of an acute post-
streptococcal glomerulonephritis.

WHAT IS THE FINAL DIAGNOSIS?

Acute glomerulonephritis (nephritic syndrome, due to a diffuse proliferative and exudative glomerulonephritis, mediated by immune
complexes), probably post-streptococcal.

HOW WOULD YOU MANAGE THIS PATIENT?

It is essential to control this patient's blood pressure. Uncontrolled
hypertension accentuates renal damage from almost any cause.
Treatment should start with a diuretic, with a beta-blocker added if
necessary. Loop diuretics will probably be needed at this level of renal
function. Should control not be achieved quickly, then a vasodilator
drug such as hydralazine or nifedipine should be added to the regimen.
Despite the low albumin, the elevated JVP implies circulatory volume
overload and there is no contraindication to using a potent loop
diuretic.

Fluid intake should be restricted to 300 ml/day until signs of fluid
overload and hypertension have resolved. Thereafter oral fluids may
be increased to 300 ml plus an allowance equal to the previous day's
output. Sodium intake should be reduced to about 40 mmol/day, which
means no added salt with food and none in the cooking. Whilst the
patient is oliguric potassium intake should be restricted to

60 mmol/day, and protein intake restricted to about 60 g/day. Further antibiotics are of no value at this stage. It is questionable whether long-term penicillin should be given prophylactically to prevent second attacks. More from tradition than from proven value, children are usually given prolonged penicillin prophylaxis:

The prognosis of this condition is so good that steroids and immunosuppressives are not usually indicated.

Progress should be monitored with daily weights, urine volumes, blood pressure and plasma creatinine. If the patient does not show signs of improvement within a week or 10 days, a repeat renal biopsy should be carried out. If the renal biopsy were to show evidence of increasing damage, it would not be unreasonable to begin immunosuppressive therapy.

COMMENT

Accurate diagnosis of glomerulonephritis must include a description of clinical syndrome, histology and aetiology.

1   *Clinical syndrome* in this patient was the nephritic syndrome of haematuria, oliguria, hypertension and impaired renal function.
2   *Histology*: the pattern of damage to the patient's glomerulus was 'a diffuse endocapillary proliferative and exudative glomerulonephritis'.
3   *Aetiology*: this patient's glomerulonephritis was an immune complex (as opposed to autoantibody) mediated disease, with the relevant antigens presumed to be derived from the beta-haemolytic *Streptococcus*.

With careful conservative management well over 80 per cent of patients make a full recovery, but a small percentage have persistent proteinuria and haematuria. It seems likely that a few of these may eventually deteriorate to end-stage chronic renal failure over the ensuing years. There is as yet insufficient evidence from prolonged follow-up to know how commonly this occurs. Prolonged follow-up should be undertaken in all patients with persistent haematuria, proteinuria, hypertension, or reduced renal function.

EXAMINERS' FOLLOW-UP QUESTIONS

1   What are the major histological types of glomerulonephritis that can be recognised by light microscopy?
2   What are the indications for steroids and/or immunosuppressive therapy in glomerulonephritis?
3   What precautions are needed before performing a renal biospy?
4   What illnesses are caused by the beta-haemolytic *Streptococcus*?
5   What is a red cell cast?

P.S.

137

Oedema

WHAT IS THE DIFFERENTIAL DIAGNOSIS?

1 Juvenile rheumatoid arthritis — Still's disease
2 Nephrotic syndrome
    Amyloidosis
    Drug-induced glomerulonephritis
    Renal vein thrombosis

The history of a deforming polyarthritis in childhood, together with the physical signs present in this man, are typical of Still's disease. Marked proteinuria and severe hypoalbuminaemia suggest the diagnosis of the nephrotic syndrome. Gross oedema can also be caused by congestive cardiac failure and advanced liver disease, but these are excluded by the absence of either a raised JVP or the stigmata of chronic liver disease. Postural hypotension and cold extremities in the presence of gross oedema imply a reduced circulating blood volume, caused by severe hypoalbuminaemia.

Amyloidosis affecting the kidney, liver, spleen and other organs is relatively common in either Still's disease or adult rheumatoid arthritis, even though the phase of active arthritis may have passed. Neither disease is associated with a specific glomerulonephritis. However, membranous glomerulonephritis can be induced by gold and penicillamine, and it may present as the nephrotic syndrome. Drug withdrawal usually leads to resolution.

Renal vein thrombosis is classically associated with loin pain, fever and haematuria, and a sudden worsening of renal function. It can, however, be remarkably silent and should be considered when a patient with the nephrotic syndrome does not respond to treatment or when renal function deteriorates unexpectedly.

WHAT ADDITIONAL INVESTIGATIONS WOULD YOU CONSIDER?

1 Urine microscopy
A fresh specimen of urine should be microscoped to detect casts. Numerous hyaline and granular casts, occasional red cells and tubular epithelial cells were found in the urine. There were no red cell casts. The finding of red cell casts is almost diagnostic of glomerulonephritis, although they are not invariably present in this condition.

2 Creatinine clearance and 24-hour urine protein excretion
This man had a creatinine clearance of 45 ml/min (normal > 90 ml/min), with 7 g proteinuria/24 hours. The urinary excretion of sodium was also measured, and found to be 2 mmol/24 hours (normal

100–300 mmol/24 h depending on diet). The patient's hypoalbumin-aemia is due to urinary loss of protein; he now has profound salt and water retention, which can be partly explained on the basis of reduced renal perfusion secondary to a reduced circulating blood volume.

3 Renal biopsy

A renal biopsy is the definitive test. It is better to mobilise some of the oedema first to make the procedure easier and less distressing for the patient. Prior to renal biopsy, coagulation studies (prothrombin time, partial thromboplastin time, thrombin time and a platelet count) should be checked. This patient's biopsy showed extensive amyloidosis, with no evidence of a glomerulonephritis. It is important to ask the histopathologist to stain biopsy material for amyloid as this is not performed routinely.

4 Cryoglobulins

Cryoglobulinaemia may occur occasionally in rheumatoid arthritis and should be excluded. This patient did not have any of the clinical features that might suggest this diagnosis (skin purpura, peripheral neuropathy, skin ulcers or Raynaud's phenomenon), and cryoglobulins were not present.

5 Immunological studies

Although less likely, an unrelated glomerulonephritis could coexist with Still's disease. It would be reasonable to measure the serum complement levels (C3 and C4), autoantibodies including antinuclear factor, DNA binding and rheumatoid factor. No abnormality was detected.

6 ECG and echocardiogram

Amyloid frequently affects the myocardium producing a congestive cardiomyopathy. Digoxin should be avoided as it may cause fatal arrhythmias. An ECG and echocardiogram were performed, but were normal.

7 Renal venogram

This investigation would be indicated if the patient failed to respond to plasma infusions and diuretics. Other indications would include loin pain and haematuria, or a sudden and unexpected worsening of renal function. Anticoagulants may preserve renal function in patients with early renal vein thrombosis; this treatable complication of the nephrotic syndrome should not be missed.

WHAT IS THE FINAL DIAGNOSIS?

Still's disease, with renal amyloidosis causing the nephrotic syndrome.

139

HOW WOULD YOU MANAGE THIS PATIENT?

Oedema of this magnitude demands treatment, which will relieve the patient's discomfort, correct any dyspnoea and prevent secondary infection.

The physical signs suggest a reduced intravascular volume. Amyloid may infiltrate the adrenal glands and produce an Addisonian state. The presence of oedema and the very low urinary sodium are strongly against adrenal insufficiency as the cause of this man's postural hypotension and poor peripheral perfusion. The very low urinary sodium may reflect intense secondary hyperaldosteronism, although other mechanisms seem likely to be responsible for avid sodium retention in the nephrotic syndrome (for example, reduced glomerular filtration rate). It should be noted that the plasma urea is considerably more elevated than the plasma creatinine. The clinical signs and this biochemistry indicate markedly impaired renal perfusion.

If large doses of a potent loop diuretic (eg frusemide) are prescribed, circulatory collapse and acute renal failure may be precipitated. This patient's oedema should be mobilised by a combination of regular intravenous albumin (50–100 ml of 20 per cent human albumin daily) together with diuretics. Diuretics should be withheld or administered with great caution until the postural hypotension and poor peripheral perfusion have been corrected. Oliguria, a rising blood urea and a very low urinary sodium are warning features of compromised renal perfusion.

The patient should be given a normal protein, low-salt diet and be restricted to 500 ml of fluid orally. Given good general nutrition, liver protein synthesis can increase markedly and the patient may be able to manage without regular protein infusions. A high protein diet is now no longer recommended in the nephrotic syndrome, as this may increase renal blood flow thereby increasing glomerular perfusion leading to an increase in proteinuria. A high protein diet does not stimulate the liver to increase protein synthesis any further.

There is no effective treatment for secondary amyloidosis. Steroids are only of value in the control of the underlying chronic inflammatory condition. Indeed, in the experimental animal steroids may accelerate the deposition of amyloid. In view of the high risk of renal vein thrombosis long-term anticoagulation with warfarin should be considered after the renal biopsy has had time to heal.

COMMENT

The nephrotic syndrome is the consequence of gross proteinuria sufficient to produce hypoproteinaemia. Glomerular filtration rate is often well preserved until intravascular volume depletion occurs or the glomerular lesion progresses to such an extent as to impair filtration. Causes include diabetes mellitus, amyloid and various forms of glomerulonephritis. A renal biopsy is virtually always required in adults to define the cause and to guide therapy. In children, the minimal change glomerular lesion is so often the cause of the nephrotic syndrome that a therapeutic trial of steroids should probably precede a biopsy.

Complications of the nephrotic syndrome include venous thrombosis (legs, iliac and renal veins) and thromboembolism. A renal vein thrombosis is a complication of the nephrotic syndrome, and not a cause.

Infection is common and may include a primary peritonitis with pneumococci, which is sometimes seen in children with a minimal change glomerular lesion.

This patient's prognosis is poor, as amyloid tends to be progressive. When cardiac amyloid develops life expectancy is limited to less than a few years. Dialysis and transplantation are possible, but these patients are particularly prone to serious infective complications.

EXAMINERS' FOLLOW-UP QUESTIONS

1   What do you know about primary peritonitis developing in patients with ascites?
2   What are the differences between the nephritic syndrome and the nephrotic syndrome?
3   What drugs may produce the nephrotic syndrome?
4   What are the other common causes of a serum albumin of 17 g/l?
5   What is the risk of hepatitis or AIDS following the use of intravenous albumin?

P.S.

Pins and needles

WHAT IS THE DIFFERENTIAL DIAGNOSIS?

1   Multiple sclerosis (MS)
    Spinal cord compression by tumour
    Transverse myelitis
    Subacute combined degeneration of the cord

Multiple sclerosis is the commonest cause of a spinal cord lesion at this age. It is suggested by the fluctuating course of the illness, and by aggravation of symptoms on exercise or neck flexion. The past history of vertigo may have been a brain stem episode.

Spinal compression must always be ruled out in any progressive paraplegia. There are many causes: extrathecal (bone disease, metastases abscess), intrathecal (meningioma, neurofibroma, astrocytoma of the cord, lymphoma). Local and radicular pain is a prominent symptom especially with extrathecal lesions. Transverse myelitis may follow viral illnesses, especially glandular fever; the onset is usually more rapid and severe than seen in this patient, and involves the whole cord. Subacute combined degeneration is unusual at this age and does not involve spinothalamic pathways.

WHAT ADDITIONAL INVESTIGATIONS WOULD YOU CONSIDER?

1   Spinal X-rays
X-rays must include both cervical and thoracic regions. They were normal.

2   Lumbar puncture
The cerebrospinal fluid was under normal pressure. The protein was 0.7 g/l (normal 0.15–0.40 g/l); 15 per cent of the total protein was IgG, with oligoclonal bands present on electrophoresis. These abnormalities are characteristic of MS.

3   Visual evoked potentials
Despite the patient's apparently normal visual function, there was prolonged latency in the cortical response to a pattern stimulus from the right eye. This indicates delayed conduction in the anterior visual pathways, in the right optic nerve. Hence, there is disseminated disease, despite the apparent localisation of disease to the spinal cord on physical examination.

142

4 Magnetic resonance imaging scan of the brain

About 50 per cent of patients with early MS, with a single clinical spinal cord lesion, show abnormal areas of high signal in the periventricular white matter.

5 Serum B12

The serum B12 was 240 mg/l (normal 160–925 mg/l) excluding subacute combined degeneration of the cord.

WHAT IS THE FINAL DIAGNOSIS?

Multiple sclerosis.

HOW WOULD YOU MANAGE THIS PATIENT?

Most acute attacks of MS progress for days or weeks, and then show spontaneous remission which may be complete. If the spinal cord disorder appears to be progressing, steroids may promote a remission although they probably do not affect long-term outlook. Prednisolone is given in a short course lasting two weeks at high dose (80 mg per day), tapering rapidly to 10 mg per day. Some workers prefer adrenocorticotrophic hormone (ACTH) injections, dexamethasone or intravenous methylprednisolone.

It is necessary to give a guarded prognosis: the patient should be advised to avoid heavy exertion, viral infections, and any immunisation procedure. Pregnancy carries a slightly increased risk of relapse.

COMMENT

The prognosis of MS is enormously variable. Poor prognosis is indicated by HLA type DrW2, frequent attacks or incomplete remission. Clinical trials of immunopressive therapy are continuing. Hyperbaric oxygen treatment has now been shown to be ineffective.

EXAMINERS' FOLLOW-UP QUESTIONS

1 Why is there such variation in the incidence of MS in different parts of the world?
2 Is optic neuritis always due to MS?
3 Can a patient complaining of urgency and incontinence of urine without symptoms in the legs be suffering from MS?
4 What measures are available for the treatment of severe spasticity and spasms in chronic MS?
5 What do you know of the theories for the cause of MS?

R.W.R.R.

Anaemia on anticoagulants

WHAT IS THE DIFFERENTIAL DIAGNOSIS?

1   Iron deficiency anaemia
       Occult gastrointestinal bleeding
           telangiectasia
           peptic ulcer
           carcinoma
           angiodysplasia of the colon

Chronic blood loss must have been present for some time judging from the marked hypochromia and microcytosis.

Over anticoagulation is likely to make itself evident by symptoms and signs such as haematuria, nose bleeds and easy bruising, none of which the patient had; in fact he had been seen at regular intervals and had been well-controlled. However, it is generally recognised that anticoagulant therapy may precipitate bleeding from some other pathology, and this often provides the very first indication of its presence.

Hereditary haemorrhagic telangiectasia is often associated with iron deficiency anaemia due to bleeding from typical lesions in the gastrointestinal tract.

The patient had no symptoms of a peptic ulcer and, at his age, it would be important to exclude a carcinoma. Angiodysplasia of the colon usually occurs in an elderly patient.

WHAT ADDITIONAL INVESTIGATIONS WOULD YOU CONSIDER?

1   Prothrombin time
Patient: 23 sec; control: 12 sec (International Normalized Ratio 2–3). His anticoagulant therapy is well-controlled.

2   Iron and total iron binding capcity
Plasma iron: 4.6 μmol/l (normal: 15–30 μmol/l)
TIBC: 64.2 μmol/l (normal: 40–70 μmol/l)
A low plasma iron and a normal iron binding capacity. The hypochromic microcytic anaemia in this patient could be due to iron deficiency or the 'anaemia of chronic disease'. Iron status is best assessed by looking at the iron stores in the bone marrow: this patient was iron deficient.

3 Faecal occult blood testing

Three stool specimens were positive for blood. The gastrointestinal tract is the most likely site for occult blood loss in any male, or post-menopausal female, who is found to have a hypochromic microcytic blood picture without haematuria.

4 Gastroscopy

Two small veins were seen at the lower end of the oesophagus but these were not varices; there was mild oesophagitis. The stomach and duodenum were normal. In particular no telangiectatic lesions were seen. Endoscopy is a more effective screen of the upper gastro-intestinal tract than a barium meal. Had the patient not been taking oral anticoagulants, the duodenum would have been biopsied (to exclude coeliac disease).

5 Barium enema

Before ordering a barium enema, the clinician must always perform a sigmoidoscopy to exclude a rectal lesion. This patient's sigmoidoscopy was normal.

'Barium flowed freely to the caecum, outlining the appendix and refluxing into the terminal ileum. There is well-marked diverticular disease of the colon, most obvious in the pelvic colon. No indication of any other abnormality.' Simple diverticular disease of the colon is not an adequate cause for occult gastrointestinal haemorrhage. The radiologist did not perform a double-contrast examination.

At this stage, with a negative gastroscopy and a negative barium study, the anticoagulant therapy could be withdrawn: regular assessment of the haemoglobin and stool testing for occult blood could be performed to see if the bleeding had stopped. In this patient it was considered that further investigation was more appropriate.

6 Colonoscopy

Two polyps were seen, one at the recto-sigmoid junction, and the second in the transverse colon; both were snared and removed. A brown polypoid nodule was seen in the ascending colon, which the endoscopist considered could be a carcinoma.

Histology of the first two polyps showed them to be tubulo-villous adenomas; the polyp from the ascending colon was a tubulo-villous adenoma with severe cytological atypia amounting to carcinoma *in situ*.

WHAT IS THE FINAL DIAGNOSIS?

Carcinoma of the colon, causing iron deficiency anaemia due to bleeding aggravated by therapeutic anticoagulation.

HOW WOULD YOU MANAGE THIS PATIENT?

The patient was admitted for laparotomy. From the time he was first seen with the hypochromic, microcytic anaemia, he had been taking ferrous sulphate; his symptoms of breathlessness on exertion had disappeared and his haemoglobin concentration was normal (13.3 g/dl). He was in excellent condition. A right hemicolectomy was performed, removing 15 cm terminal ileum and 21 cm of the ascending colon; no secondary deposits were noted. Histology showed that the tumour was a moderately differentiated mucin-secreting adenocarcinoma, infiltrating the bowel wall through to the serosa. The resection margins were free of tumour and the five lymph nodes that were examined were clear of tumour; no blood vessels were involved. The conclusion was adenocarcinoma of the colon, Dukes' stage B.

COMMENT

Frank blood loss in a patient on oral anticoagulant drugs usually poses few problems in diagnosis. With occult bleeding, one needs to be satisfied that the patient's anticoagulation is not out of control; an excessively prolonged prothrombin time could reflect some change in the patient's own physical condition, or the coincident use of another drug (eg aspirin, cimetidine or antibiotic) which leads to a higher free level of the anticoagulant.

Patients with telangiectasia often have very troublesome bleeding from their vascular malformations; this patient was not even aware of the lesions in his mouth, but he would have noticed if they were bleeding. Lesions lower down the gastrointestinal tract could easily have bled and produced the iron deficiency anaemia.

At this patient's age, one must be quite satisfied that there is not another pathology which is being declared by the anticoagulant therapy. The negative barium studies posed an additional, but not uncommon, hazard for this type of patient. He was known to be bleeding from the gastrointestinal tract, yet the barium enema was negative. Knowing the problem, the radiologist might modify the technique to concentrate attention to certain sites or suggest another investigation, for example, gastrointestinal angiography.

Problem gastrointestinal haemorrhage in the elderly, either occult or overt, is often due to angiodysplasia — abnormal submucosal blood vessels mostly found in the caecum or right colon. These vessels can only be detected by aggressive investigation such as colonoscopy or angiography.

EXAMINERS' FOLLOW-UP QUESTIONS

1 Should this patient have follow-up colonoscopy examinations?
2 What commonly-used drugs may affect anticoagulation?
3 What would you do about his anticoagulant therapy prior to surgery?
4 How may angiodysplasia of the colon be treated?
5 Why may a right hemicolectomy cause troublesome diarrhoea?

E.J.P.-W.

'Pains in all my joints'

WHAT IS THE DIFFERENTIAL DIAGNOSIS?

1   Rheumatoid arthritis
    Carcinoma of the lung
    Tuberculosis

Joint swelling associated with tenderness and early morning stiffness is strongly suggestive of an inflammatory arthritis. The widespread symmetrical involvement of both large and small joints is best compatible with a diagnosis of rheumatoid arthritis. Hypertrophic pulmonary osteoarthropathy may occasionally produce sufficient periarticular pain and synovitis to mimic early rheumatoid arthritis. The signs of a pleural effusion are compatible with a complication of rheumatoid arthritis, but an additional local problem must be excluded. The muscle wasting and weakness in the hands suggest compression of the median nerve.

WHAT ADDITIONAL INVESTIGATIONS WOULD YOU CONSIDER?

1 Rheumatoid factor
This was demonstrated by agglutination of latex particles coated with human immunoglobulin, and found to be positive at a titre of 1:320. This test has a 70–80 per cent sensitivity in rheumatoid arthritis, but poor specificity, as the production of rheumatoid factors has been associated with many other diseases with autoallergic features.

2 Hand and feet X-rays
In the hands there was slight periarticular osteoporosis. There was a small erosion in the 3rd metatarsophalangeal joint. There was no periostitis. It is common in rheumatoid arthritis for the earliest erosions to appear in the feet. It is unusual for erosions to develop within six months of the onset of disease.

3 Chest X-ray
This confirmed the right-sided pleural effusion. There was no apparent mass lesion and the cardiac size was normal.

4 Pleural aspirate
Diagnostic aspirate of the pleural space produced a clear yellow liquid. Analysis of this showed a protein concentration of 45 g/l (an exudate rather than a transudate); the glucose was 1.8 mmol/l; latex was positive and acid-fast bacilli were not present; cytology showed only polymorphs in the fluid.

5   Schirmer's test

Using a standard commercial strip of filter paper in each eye, 7 mm of wetting was seen at five minutes (normal > 15 mm). This is evidence of keratoconjunctivitis sicca (part of the triad of Sjögren's syndrome). Features of Sjögren's syndrome are found in up to 30 per cent of patients with rheumatoid arthritis.

6   Nerve conduction studies and electromyography

Muscle sampling of both abductor pollicis brevis muscles showed the pattern of 'chronic partial devervation'. Nerve conduction studies showed prolonged distal latencies and reduced sensory action potentials in both median nerves. The changes confirm the clinical diagnosis of bilateral carpal tunnel syndrome. In this patient the clinical grounds for suspecting this common complication of rheumatoid arthritis were high, and this fairly time-consuming test was not really necessary.

WHAT IS THE FINAL DIAGNOSIS?

Seropositive erosive rheumatoid arthritis, with a pleural effusion and bilateral carpal tunnel syndrome.

HOW WOULD YOU MANAGE THIS PATIENT?

The patient has both clinical and laboratory signs of continuing disease activity. Basic management includes rest during periods of active disease, splints, and physiotherapy. Drug therapy should include non-steroidal anti-inflammatory agents. Symptoms of carpal tunnel compression often respond well to local steroid injections though surgical decompression may ultimately be required. Intra-articular steroid injections to a few severely affected joints, especially knee and shoulders, may provide considerable symptomatic relief.

This patient has persistent and progressive disease with evidence of erosions only six months after the onset of symptoms. It would be current practice in most units also to introduce 'second-line' drugs at this stage. The choice lies between gold, penicillamine hydroxy-chloroquine and, in severe cases, methotrexate.

Corticosteroids are in general contraindicated in uncomplicated rheumatoid arthritis but, in doses of less than 10 mg of prednisolone daily, they may provide good relief for patients with persistently active synovitis refractory to other treatments. Oral corticosteroid therapy is often necessary to control extra-articular complications of rheumatoid arthritis including vasculitis, pulmonary involvement and Felty's syndrome. In this patient prednisolone 10 mg nocte slowed reaccumulation of the pleural fluid, and it was possible to reduce the daily dose to 6 mg. Azathioprine is reserved for those with severe systemic disease, or it is used as a steroid-sparing agent.

COMMENT

It is unusual for rheumatoid arthritis to progress relentlessly. Most patients will receive pain relief from non-steroidal anti-inflammatory agents, although it may be necessary to try several at full dosage before finding a preparation that agrees with the patient.

Diagnosis of respiratory problems in patients with rheumatoid arthritis may be very difficult. It is usually necessary to exclude second diagnoses before attributing pulmonary or pleural disease to the rheumatoid process.

EXAMINERS' FOLLOW-UP QUESTIONS

1　What are the hand deformities of rheumatoid arthritis?
2　What other pulmonary complications of rheumatoid arthritis may occur?
3　What are the side-effects of gold therapy?
4　How do the radiological features of osteoarthritis differ from those of rheumatoid arthritis?
5　What do you know about therapy with gold by mouth?

M.J.W.
G.R.V.H.

Loin pain and fever

WHAT IS THE DIFFERENTIAL DIAGNOSIS?

1 Septicaemia
   Acute left pyelonephritis
2 Renal vein thrombosis
3 Arterial embolus to the left kidney
4 Neurogenic bladder
   Spina bifida occulta
5 Pregnancy, possibly ectopic
6 Longstanding renal impairment
   Chronic pyelonephritis

The clinical picture is that of a severe bacterial infection producing a septicaemia. She is flushed and hypotensive; the high leucocyte count supports the diagnosis of bacterial infection. From the history and the physical findings of loin pain and tenderness, the source of this infection is almost certainly the urinary tract.

This unfortunate young girl has two good reasons for developing an acute upper urinary tract infection. During pregnancy hormonal changes relax smooth muscles: a considerable degree of ureteric dilatation occurs and free vesico-ureteric reflux is not uncommon. Bladder emptying is also impaired. In pregnancy about 25 per cent of lower urinary tract infections ascend and develop into full-blown acute pyelonephritis, as in this patient. In addition to pregnancy, her history of enuresis and the neurological abnormalities suggest sacral nerve root lesions, which are compatible with a diagnosis of spina bifida. Rectal examination may reveal a patulous anus with poor sphincter tone. Sensation in the saddle area is often impaired. Destruction of the sacral nerve roots impairs the nerve supply to the bladder. A poorly emptying neurogenic bladder predisposes to urinary tract infection and increases the risk of ascending infection.

A lower abdominal mass, amenorrhoea and sudden hypotensive collapse could be due to a ruptured ectopic pregnancy. Fever and leucocytosis would also be compatible with this diagnosis. However, the loin pain, tenderness and fullness point very strongly to a renal pathology.

An arterial embolus will produce acute loin pain and haematuria. Neither the history nor the examination suggests a source for the embolus. Unless there were bilateral emboli, a raised urea and creatinine would be unlikely as the other kidney would probably be normal.

A renal vein thrombosis may occur in patients who are dehydrated, or who are prone to thrombotic complications (eg pregnancy or the oral contraceptive pill). It may also complicate pre-existing renal disease (eg the nephrotic syndrome due to membranous glomerulonephritis or amyloidosis). The sudden onset of this illness in a previously fit young girl makes a renal thrombosis unlikely.

At this stage it is difficult to be sure what this girl's renal function was like before she became ill. The raised urea and creatinine could be due to impaired renal perfusion (pre-renal) with the septicaemia. The haemoglobin of 10.8 g/dl could suggest chronic disease, but the anaemia could be due to haemolysis during severe septicaemia (a normal bilirubin is against this). The long history of lower urinary tract symptoms suggest recurrent infections during childhood. Long-standing chronic pyelonephritis, due to the reflux of infected urine, is therefore likely.

WHAT ADDITIONAL INVESTIGATIONS WOULD YOU CONSIDER?

1 Microbiology
Urine and blood cultures should be taken immediately before any anti-biotics are started. As she is clinically toxic with vasodilatation and hypotension, it is likely that a blood culture will be positive, but bacterial sensitivities will not be available for 48 hours. The blood and urine cultures grew E. coli.

2 Differential white blood cell count
The clinical impression of a severe bacterial infection was supported by finding a 92 per cent neutrophilia in the differential white blood cell count.

3 Pregnancy test
This was positive.

4 Urgent abdominal ultrasound
Abdominal X-rays should not be taken because of the suspected pregnancy. An ultrasound of the kidneys showed a small scarred right kidney and some focal loss of renal tissue from the upper pole of the left kidney. There was no evidence of obstruction. Abdominal ultrasound confirmed the presence of a gravid uterus.

5 Assessment of renal function
After resolution of the acute episode more detailed investigations should be undertaken. Her creatinine clearance was 35 ml/min when measured two months after her acute illness (normal 90–120 ml/min). Given the expected increase in glomerular filtration that normally occurs in pregnancy this represents quite advanced renal damage. Her 24-hour urinary protein excretion was 400 mg/24 hours which is compatible with chronic pyelonephritis.

6 Intravenous pyelogram

A high-dose IVP was carried out two months after delivery. This showed persistent slight dilatation of the ureters in keeping with the history of a urinary tract infection during pregnancy. Although this dilatation usually resolves, it may not do so, and by itself does not necessarily mean obstruction. The left kidney showed focal loss of cortex in the upper pole, with clubbing of the underlying calyces. The right kidney showed extensive scarring, with loss of cortex and distortion of both upper and lower pole calyces. These are the typical radiological features of advanced chronic pyelonephritis. The bladder was thin-walled and large. It did not contract well, as the after-micturition film showed a large residue. Spina bifida was noted. These findings are in keeping with an atonic (lower motor neurone type) neurogenic bladder.

7 Micturating cysto-urethrogram

The bladder required 950 ml of contrast to fill it (most female bladders will only hold up to 500 ml). There was free reflux up the right ureter to the kidney. There was a lesser degree of reflux on the left side. Bladder contraction was poor and there was a large residual volume of contrast in the bladder.

WHAT IS THE FINAL DIAGNOSIS?

Acute pyelonephritis with an associated *E. coli* septicaemia. Moderate chronic renal failure due to chronic pyelonephritis caused by vesico-ureteric reflux from a neurogenic bladder (spina bifida occulta).

HOW WOULD YOU MANAGE THIS PATIENT?

This young girl is acutely ill with a serious bacterial infection. There is a risk of abortion. After blood and urine cultures have been taken she should be started immediately on parenteral antibiotics. Most urinary tract infections are due to bowel organisms, unless instrumentation has occurred. Parenteral ampicillin or cefotaxime would cover most common urinary pathogens.

In addition to chemotherapy this girl needs volume expansion with parenteral fluids. She is vasodilated and hypotensive, and may therefore require as much as four to six litres of intravenous fluids over the first 24 hours. The first litre (0.9 per cent saline) should be given quickly over an hour, and the subsequent rate of infusion determined by her clinical response.

Parenteral antibiotics may need to be continued for two or three days. The dose of cefotaxime was reduced to two-thirds of normal after three days, as her renal function did not improve despite rehydration. It is essential to continue with antibiotics for a prolonged period. Loin pain and tenderness should resolve completely, and the treatment be continued for a further week. Serial midstream urine cultures must be performed after cessation of chemotherapy, to ensure that the infection has been completely eradicated. Continued careful ante-natal follow-up is essential. Long-term prophylactic antibiotics should be considered. If bladder emptying is grossly impaired, self-catheterisations every four to six hours can be helpful.

COMMENT

The distinction between acute pyelonephritis and chronic pyelonephritis is important as the terminology is poor. Acute pyelonephritis is a sudden severe acute infection of the upper urinary tract with pus and bacteria within the renal pelvis, calyces or collecting ducts of the kidney. Untreated acute pyelonephritis spreads into the renal parenchyma with tissue destruction, and septicaemia is not uncommon. Effective antibacterial therapy will eradicate the infection and is usually associated with preservation of renal function. It is essential that treatment be continued until all renal tenderness has settled, which usually means at least two to three weeks of full antibacterial therapy.

Chronic pyelonephritis, on the other hand, is really a radiological diagnosis (cortical scarring, plus calcyceal distortion or clubbing). It usually presents in young adult life with hypertension and impaired renal function. At this time both the urine and kidney tissue are sterile. In most patients the disease originates during infancy, when infection from the lower urinary tract ascends because of vesico-ureteric reflux. An insidious and progressive scarring develops which continues long after the eradication of any identifiable bacteria in the urine. The mechanism of this progressive scarring is not known.

EXAMINERS' FOLLOW-UP QUESTIONS

1 What may be done to reduce the incidence of chronic pyelonephritis?
2 Under what circumstances would you advise reimplantation of the ureters?
3 Which antibacterial agents would you avoid in pregnancy, and why?
4 What other infections may present with rigors?
5 Which of the 'screening tests' have different normal ranges in pregnancy?

P.S.

Pruritus for six months

WHAT IS THE DIFFERENTIAL DIAGNOSIS?

1   Primary biliary cirrhosis
    Primary sclerosing cholangitis
    Choledocholithiasis
    Drug-related cholestasis

The slow onset of itching in a middle-aged woman with serum bio-chemical tests suggesting mild cholestasis strongly support the diagnosis of primary biliary cirrhosis (chronic non-suppurative intra-hepatic cholangitis). The association with goitre and rheumatoid arthritis supports the diagnosis. Sclerosing cholangitis is less likely in view of the absence of ulcerative colitis, or the febrile symptoms of bacterial cholangitis.

Choledocholithiasis is also unlikely in the absence of episodes of biliary pain and fever.

Drug-related cholestasis due, for instance, to chlorpromazine or to sex hormones, is unlikely in view of the absence of a history of drug ingestion.

WHAT ADDITIONAL INVESTIGATIONS WOULD YOU CONSIDER?

1   Serum autoantibodies

If correctly performed, the serum mitochondrial antibody test is positive in 98 per cent of patients with primary biliary cirrhosis. A negative result throws the diagnosis into doubt and necessitates other investigations. In this patient, it was positive in a titre exceeding 1:40. The explanation for a positive result is unknown: it is not related to aetiology.

2   Serum immunoglobulins

Serum IgM is usually increased in primary biliary cirrhosis and, if so, supports the diagnosis. In this patient the value was 4.0 g/l (normal 0.6–2.8 g/l).

3   Endoscopic retrograde cholangiopancreatography

This showed a normal common bile duct and intrahepatic ducts. This excluded the diagnosis of primary sclerosing cholangitis where irregular intra-hepatic and extra-hepatic bile ducts are seen. Gallstones in the gall-bladder are frequently associated with primary biliary cirrhosis, but none were found in this patient. If the endoscopist had failed to cannulate into the biliary tree, percutaneous cholangiography may be used to visualise the bile ducts and prove that they are normal.

4 Liver biopsy

Before this test is performed, the prothrombin time must be restored to normal by intramuscular vitamin K1. In this patient, the histological picture was of a stage I primary biliary cirrhosis, with damage to the epithelium of small ducts in the liver and surrounding granuloma formation. The lobular structure of the liver was normal and cirrhosis was not present. In spite of its name, a true nodular cirrhosis is a very late feature of primary biliary cirrhosis.

The liver biopsy was most important for this patient: it confirmed the diagnosis and showed that the disease was at an early stage. In addition, the presence of granulomas makes the prognosis much better.

5 Upper gastrointestinal endoscopy (or barium swallow)

Either procedure can be used to establish the presence or absence of oesophageal varices. In this patient they were absent.

6 Serum cholesterol

This is usually normal in the early stages of the disease. This patient's serum cholesterol was 9.2 mmol/l (normal 3.0–6.5 mmol/l).

WHAT IS THE FINAL DIAGNOSIS?

Primary biliary cirrhosis.

HOW WOULD YOU MANAGE THIS PATIENT?

The outlook for this patient with very early disease is unpredictable, except that the disease is not curable at present. However, she may stay in her present state for a great many years. The presence of granulomas on the liver biopsy and the absence of jaundice are good prognostic features. The patient should be reassured, and she and her family instilled with a spirit of optimism. She should lead a normal life.

In spite of the absence of jaundice no harm will be done by attempting to prevent the complications of prolonged cholestasis, which include the effects of steatorrhoea. The fat-soluble vitamins A (100 000 units), D (100 000 units) and K1 (10 mg) should be given intra-muscularly every four weeks. Vitamin E 200 mg daily orally is useful although deficiency of this vitamin is unusual except in those with deep jaundice. She should encourage vitamin D synthesis in the skin by sunshine and, in temperate climates in the winter, by an ultra-violet lamp. Skimmed milk is a useful calcium supplement.

Pruritus is controlled by cholestyramine in a dose usually between 8 and 16 g daily, taken before meals.

There is no satisfactory treatment for primary biliary cirrhosis. The most recent is ursodeoxycholic acid which may act as a choleretic flushing out toxic bile acids.

COMMENT

Primary biliary cirrhosis is being increasingly diagnosed with greater awareness of the significance of a raised serum alkaline phosphatase value in a woman. Diagnosis is being made earlier and the prognosis is correspondingly much better. In the asymptomatic patient the outlook is the same as for any other woman of the same age. The advanced stages of the disease are marked by deepening of cholestatic jaundice, the development of skin xanthomas, osteomalacia and ultimately liver failure with ascites, hepatic encephalopathy and terminal bleeding from oesophageal varices.

EXAMINERS' FOLLOW-UP QUESTIONS

1 What are the theories for the cause of the intrahepatic bile duct damage in primary biliary cirrhosis?
2 What possible later complications may this patient show?
3 What precautions should you take when prescribing cholestyramine?
4 Can the results of liver function tests be used in patients with primary biliary cirrhosis, to assess prognosis?
5 Should patients with primary biliary cirrhosis be considered for hepatic transplantation and what results can be expected?

S.S.

Recurrent chest infections

WHAT IS THE DIFFERENTIAL DIAGNOSIS?

1 Chronic lymphocytic leukaemia
2 Recurrent chest infections
   Hypogammaglobulinaemia
   Neutropenia
   Defects of cellular immune responses
   Tuberculosis
   Bronchiectasis
   Carcinoma
3 Anaemia and purpura
   Marrow infiltration
   Immune haemolysis and thrombocytopenia
   Hypersplenism

The combination of recurrent chest infections and chronic lymphocytic leukaemia is very suggestive of hypogammaglobulinaemia, but opportunistic infections in a patient with a malignant disease should always be considered.

For many patients with chronic lymphocytic leukaemia, especially the symptomatic variety, the development of a pancytopenia is often an indication that bone marrow failure is occurring. Other complications, such as autoimmune blood disorders, need to be excluded.

WHAT ADDITIONAL INVESTIGATIONS WOULD YOU CONSIDER?

1 Chest radiograph
'Compared to the previous chest X-ray, there is now consolidation in the left lower lobe, with a small left pleural effusion. The appearances suggest an active infection.'

The earlier examination had shown shadowing at both lung bases, which appeared to be largely interstitial; two main possibilities for this change were considered: either a drug reaction or infection.

Cytotoxic drugs are known to cause interstitial fibrosis. Busulphan is perhaps the best-known drug causing this type of lung pathology; it is a rare complication of chlorambucil therapy, so an infection is much more likely.

2 Serum immunoglobulins
IgA: 0.3 g/l (normal 0.5–4.0 g/l)
IgG: 2.1 g/l (normal 5.0–15 g/l)
IgM: 0.4 g/l (normal 0.6–2.8 g/l)

A protein electrophoretic strip showed a marked decrease in the gammaglobulin region, and the reduced concentrations of all classes of serum immunoglobulin confirm that observation. Most patients with progressive chronic lymphocytic leukaemia can be expected to become hypogammaglobulinaemic. A paraprotein is found in the serum of a small proportion of these patients (3 to 5%) and may sometimes be associated with symptoms due to hyperviscosity or cryoprecipitation.

3 Sputum culture
Mucopurulent sputum was obtained, and a very scanty growth of *Haemophilus influenzae* was isolated. No alcohol/acid-fast bacilli were seen on microscopy and *Mycobacterium tuberculosis* was not isolated on culture.

The common infective organisms, such as *H. influenzae* or the *Pneumococcus*, are still the most likely agents. However, in a patient with a malignant blood disorder, infection with tuberculosis, a fungus, or a protozoon (such as *Pneumocystis carinii*) should be considered, particularly if there is a poor response to conventional antibiotic therapy.

4 Blood count, film, and reticulocyte count
Total white cell count: 47.8 × 10^9/l (normal 4–11 × 10^9/l)
Differential white cell count: neutrophils 14 per cent, lymphocytes 85 per cent, monocytes 1 per cent
Total neutrophil count: 6.7 × 10^9/l (normal 2–7.5 × 10^9/l)
Platelet count: 36 × 10^9/l (normal 140–400 × 10^9/l)
Reticulocytes: 3.6 per cent
There was a slight left shift in the neutrophils which also showed toxic granulation. He was mounting a reasonable neutrophil response to the infection, and neutropenia is an unlikely reason for the recurrent chest infections.

The reduced platelet count could be due to a number of causes, such as the prolonged use of cytoxic drugs, increasing leukaemic infiltration of the bone marrow or hypersplenism. In some patients an autoimmune thrombocytopenia develops: the platelet count is usually profoundly reduced with this complication, and there is marked purpura with spontaneous bleeding.

The normochromic anaemia could be caused by any of the mechanisms described for the thrombocytopenia. Although the reticulocyte count is 3.6 per cent this is not raised as the haemoglobin is only 9.8 g/dl; this suggests that reduced red cell survival is not an important factor in the anaemia. The anaemia is more likely to be due to reduced cell production.

5 Direct Coombs' test
Negative. An autoimmune haemolytic anaemia, with a positive Coombs' test, develops in about 10 per cent of patients with chronic lymphocytic leukaemia.

6 Bone marrow

Small, densely packed particles were obtained, consisting mainly of mature lymphocytes, though there was some evidence of pleomorphism. Erythroid, granulocytic and megakaryocytic elements were all present, seemingly in adequate numbers.

The aspiration of bone marrow particles may be quite difficult in chronic lymphocytic leukaemia because of the degree of infiltration. To stage this leukaemia a bone marrow trephine biopsy is usually performed, but it does not really alter the impression given by the examination of aspirated marrow particles.

This bone marrow established that the anaemia and thrombocytopenia are not due to a lack of precursor cells, but they are almost certainly related to the amount of lymphocytic infiltration in the bone marrow.

WHAT IS THE FINAL DIAGNOSIS?

Chronic lymphocytic leukaemia, with hypogammaglobulinaemia causing recurrent chest infections, and anaemia and thrombocytopenia due to bone marrow infiltration.

HOW WOULD YOU MANAGE THIS PATIENT?

The acute chest infection should be treated with a broad-spectrum antibiotic, for example erythromycin 500 mg qds together with physiotherapy and postural drainage. Unfortunately, within a few days he developed an *E. coli* urinary tract infection with septicaemia, which was treated with cefotaxime lg eight-hourly.

The patient's main problem is his increased susceptibility to infection. With the virtual absence of immunoglobulins, gammaglobulin replacement therapy is necessary. Because of his thrombocytopenia, this cannot be given intramuscularly, as each large injection would cause a muscle haematoma. He should be started on regular infusions of intravenous immunoglobulin to maintain the immunoglobin concentration within the normal range. In addition, he should receive alternating weekly courses of cotrimoxazole and doxycycline.

COMMENT

The disease in this patient shows a progression of complications due to infection and increasing marrow infiltration. The latter will lead eventually to pancytopenia and the features of bone marrow failure. Intravenous immunoglobulin is very expensive. A cheap and reasonable alternative is fresh frozen plasma, two units every week.

The mean survival of patients with chronic lymphocytic leukaemia is about five years, but there are patients who live for more than 15 years after the diagnosis has been made and die from unrelated causes. Unlike chronic granulocytic leukaemia, it is very rare for chronic lymphocytic leukaemia to progress to acute leukaemia; the usual cause of death from the disease is either infection or bone marrow failure.

EXAMINERS' FOLLOW-UP QUESTIONS

1 How could you treat immune thrombocytopenia in chronic lymphocytic leukaemia?
2 Should a patient with chronic lymphocytic leukaemia receive smallpox vaccination?
3 How would you manage *Herpes zoster* infection in this patient?
4 What hazards are associated with intravenous gentamicin?
5 What are the various stages of chronic lymphocytic leukaemia and how does this relate to survival?

E.J.P.-W

A confused patient

WHAT IS THE DIFFERENTIAL DIAGNOSIS?

1 Polycythaemia
   Polycythaemia rubra vera
   Secondary polycythaemia
      Cerebellar haemangioma
      Kidney tumour/cyst
   Relative polycythaemia
   Smokers' polycythaemia
2 Meningitis

The history and the physical findings, together with the increase in the haemoglobin and white cell count, would be highly suggestive of poly-cythaemia rubra vera, although the presentation is unusual. However, the possibility of a relative polycythaemia, perhaps due to the vomiting associated with meningism, has to be entertained. An absolute secondary polycythaemia likewise has to be considered, especially as he could have a brain tumour that had bled. Lung pathology may need to be excluded as he was a heavy smoker.

WHAT ADDITIONAL INVESTIGATIONS WOULD YOU CONSIDER?

1 Spinal tap and examination of the cerebrospinal fluid
The CSF was colourless and contained 10 red cells and five white cells × 10^6/l; the CSF protein and sugar were normal. Subsequent culture of the CSF was sterile.

2 Blood film examination
A good blood film was difficult to make, and the film appeared 'packed', meaning that the blood was too thick to spread properly. The red cells were hypochromic and microcytic; there was a neutrophil leucocytosis, with a few metamyelocytes and an increased number of basophils. Platelets were increased on the blood film, an impression confirmed by the platelet count (540 × 10^9/l). There was an increase in all the mature blood cells which, with the basophilia, is very sugges-tive of polycythaemia rubra vera. In the secondary or relative poly-cythaemias only an erythrocytosis is evident.

3 Red cell and plasma volume
Using the patient's own red cells, labelled with radioactive chromium (^{51}Cr), and radioiodinated human serum albumin (^{125}I), the following figures were obtained:
Red cell volume: 58.2 ml/kg (normal: 30 ± 3 ml/kg)

Plasma volume: 42.1 ml/kg (normal: 45 ± 5 ml/kg)
Total blood volume: 100.3 ml/kg (normal: 70 ± 5 ml/kg)
This study shows a raised red cell volume and a normal plasma volume, but it does not distinguish between a primary and secondary polycythaemia. It certainly rules out a relative polycythaemia, where the only abnormality would be a reduced plasma volume.

4 Blood gas analysis
Normal values were obtained. The presence of arterial hypoxaemia is found in those secondary polycythaemias associated with lung abnormalities. The fact that his lips were cyanosed does not indicate central hypoxia; this sign is due to hyperviscosity slowing circulation through the surface capillaries.

5 Abdominal ultrasound
No abnormality was seen in the kidneys. The liver and spleen were enlarged but the echogenic pattern was normal. In those patients where the diagnosis is clearly polycythaemia rubra vera, this examination is not necessary. In a patient with secondary polycythaemia it is important to exclude an erythropoietin-producing kidney tumour or cyst as these are the more common causes of this condition (but less common than secondary polycythaemia caused by smoking, cardiac or respiratory disease). Likewise, hepatomas can produce erythropoietin and cause a secondary polycythaemia. If an abnormal kidney is demonstrated, this should be investigated by an intravenous urogram, and possibly an arteriogram if a tumour is discovered.

6 Bone marrow
A hypercellular sample was aspirated, with a generalised increase of all the haemopoietic elements; megakaryocytes were especially prominent. Perhaps the only reason for doing a bone marrow would be to show that there was not just an erythroid hyperplasia (the hallmark of a secondary polycythaemia).

7 Neutrophil alkaline phosphatase
The score after counting 100 consecutive neutrophils was 136. Each neutrophil staining reaction is scored from zero to four and the normal range for the total score is from 15 to 100. This raised neutrophil alkaline phosphatase score supports a diagnosis of polycythaemia rubra vera. In secondary polycythaemia the score is normal, unless there is some other reason for a neutrophilia — for example, infection or tumour breakdown.

8 Serum vitamin B12 concentration
The vitamin B12 level was 1577 ng/l (normal 160–925 ng/l). Granulocytes produce transcobalamin I, one of the vitamin B12-binding proteins. An increased level of this protein has been recognised in patients with a high neutrophil count, as in a response to infection or in

such conditions as granulocytic leukaemia or polycythaemia rubra vera.

This investigation is not of major importance, although a raised vitamin B12 level can be used as a positive factor to distinguish primary from secondary polycythaemia.

9 Haemoglobin electrophoresis
No abnormal haemoglobin was demonstrated. An unnecessary test for this patient, but where there is nothing else left to suggest a cause for secondary polycythaemia, it may be of value. It may reveal an abnormal haemoglobin in which the oxygen affinity is increased four to six fold. A family history of polycythaemia, or the complications of a high haemoglobin level, may be relevant.

WHAT IS THE FINAL DIAGNOSIS?

Polycythaemia rubra vera.

HOW WOULD YOU MANAGE THIS PATIENT?

The danger of not treating this patient with some urgency is that he might suffer a major cerebrovascular catastrophe. Already it is clear that, with the increased blood viscosity, his cerebral circulation is being compromised, perhaps aggravated by atherosclerotic changes. He had to be sedated because of his agitated state. An urgent programme of venesections was started the night he came into hospital, before the diagnosis was completely established. At first, fluid replacement was given so as not to reduce the circulating blood volume too quickly. Over the next four days, two litres of blood were removed, resulting in a complete return to rational behaviour. Frequent venesections were required to keep the packed cell volume below 0.45.

During the ensuing months the platelet count rose to over $1000 \times 10^9/l$. Myelosuppressive therapy was indicated and 5mCi radioactive phosphorus (^{32}P) was given intravenously; this reduced the platelet count to $180 \times 10^9/l$; the need for venesections decreased. The frequency of ^{32}P injections, or the need to use them, varies from patient to patient. The aim is to maintain the packed red cell volume below 0.45 and to take action if the platelets increase too much.

Chemotherapy is an alternative to ^{32}P. Chlorambucil can be used to control all elements of the bone marrow, or busulphan if it is necessary to control only the platelet count.

COMMENT

Polycythaemia rubra vera is a chronic disease and, if left untreated, will lead to thrombotic or haemorrhagic complications and death within two years in 50 per cent of patients. The outlook in the well-controlled patient is very good, particularly if one remembers that it is a condition seen mainly in the older patient. Many patients survive longer than 12 years from diagnosis.

Polycythaemia rubra vera is one of the myeloproliferative group of diseases and a clonal nature has been demonstrated. After some years, with regular venesections and perhaps myelosuppressive therapy to control the disease, it often passes through a relatively quiet phase and then undergoes a change to one of the other disorders in this group, such as myelofibrosis or acute granulocytic leukaemia. A regular watch should be maintained on the clinical and laboratory features, so that these changes can be recognised.

Recent evidence suggests that cerebral blood flow is quite sensitive to the level of the packed red cell volume and, if this is kept below 0.45, delivery of oxygen is improved. With repeated venesection, the cells will become more hypochromic and microcytic and the red cell deformability may be decreased — a balance has to be achieved.

EXAMINERS' FOLLOW-UP QUESTIONS

1 What is stress polycythaemia?
2 Would a carbonmonoxyhaemoglobin measurement be of value? If so, when around you collect the sample?
3 Is there any contraindication to the use of ^{32}P or chlorambucil?
4 What causes the skin irritation?
5 Is surgery a hazard for a patient with polycythaemia rubra vera?

E.J.P.-W.

A Chelsea pensioner

WHAT IS THE DIFFERENTIAL DIAGNOSIS?

1   Chronic bronchitis and emphysema
     Cor pulmonale
   Chronic pulmonary embolism
     Pulmonary hypertension
   Bronchial carcinoma
     Lymphangitis carcinomatosa
   Alveolar cell carcinoma.

The most likely diagnosis must be increasing severity of chronic bronchitis and cor pulmonale, due to an acute respiratory infection. The elevated neck veins, hepatomegaly and peripheral oedema indicate secondary heart failure or cor pulmonale. He breathes with pursed-lip expiration in an attempt to prevent airways collapse and air trapping; he maintains an elevated intrathoracic pressure by exhaling slowly against the pursed lips which raises the oral or intralaryngeal pressure. The bounding pulse, flapping tremor, and eye signs all suggest carbon dioxide retention.

The remaining items in the differential diagnosis are much less common causes for this type of deterioration in a chronic bronchitic who smokes.

WHAT ADDITIONAL INVESTIGATIONS WOULD YOU CONSIDER?

1 Arterial blood gases
He had a low arterial oxygen (PaO_2 7.5 kPa (56 mmHg)) which has caused the compensatory polycythaemia. The clinical suspicion of carbon dioxide retention was confirmed by elevation of the arterial PCO_2 (6.6 kPa (50 mmHg)), which led to a compensated respiratory acidosis (pH 7.32).

2 ECG
The ECG showed changes of right ventricular hypertrophy: there was an R wave greater than 7 mm in V1; the combined voltage of the R wave in V1 and the S wave V6 was more than 10 mm; the R wave was taller than the S wave in V6.

3 Lung function tests
He was too distressed for any but the simplest bedside tests; his peak flow was 100 l/min. He was unable to blow out a match with his mouth wide open, indicating considerable air flow obstruction. This match

166

trick is the poor man's measurement of peak expiratory flow (but remember to switch off the oxygen cylinder before doing the trick).

4   Chest X-ray
The chest X-ray showed hyperinflation, low flat diaphragms, a deep postero-anterior diameter, loss of the retrosternal air space, and a little fluid at both costophrenic angles. There was no sign of either pneumonia or carcinoma. The appearances were those of chronic bronchitis, with emphysema.

WHAT IS THE FINAL DIAGNOSIS?

Chronic bronchitis and emphysema, causing cor pulmonale.

HOW WOULD YOU MANAGE THIS PATIENT?

He needs diuretics and metered oxygen to correct the congestive cardiac failure and the low oxygen saturation. Hypoxaemia is the more important problem, and he should receive oxygen using a 28 per cent Ventimask. The blood gases should be repeated after two hours to check that the PCO_2 is not rising. Oral frusemide (40 mg) will probably be sufficient to initiate a diuresis.

As the patient has purulent sputum he should be treated with an antibiotic such as ampicillin or oxytetracycline. A sample of the sputum should be sent for culture, and the antibiotic may be later changed when the results are available. Were the patient to be more seriously ill, a combination of parenteral ampicillin, flucloxacillin and benzyl penicillin would cover most pulmonary pathogens.

Bronchodilator drugs are sometimes beneficial: he may be helped by nebulised salbutamol (2.5 ml of a 0.5 per cent solution, six-hourly).

In his present state he does not feel like smoking, which is just as well. As he improves, he must not be allowed to restart smoking. If necessary, the smoking habit may be overcome by the help of nicotine chewing gum or hypnosis.

When he is fit for discharge, domiciliary ambulatory oxygen will help to keep him going, and a home oxygen concentrator may also be worthwhile. He should be given a supply of a broad-spectrum antibiotic, so that he can start treatment himself within hours of developing either an upper respiratory infection, or a change in the colour of his sputum.

COMMENT

Chronic bronchitis is due to hypertrophy of the bronchial mucus glands with variable mucociliary clearance. These changes lead to permanent limitation of expiratory air flow, hyperinflation of the lungs and finally impairment of gas exchange.

Emphysema is present when there is enlargement of air spaces beyond the terminal bronchioles, with destruction of lung tissue. Smoking recruits alveolar macrophages to liberate a chemotactic factor which attracts neutrophils to the lungs. This sequence induces pulmonary elastase to destroy the elastic tissue of the lungs, leading to emphysema.

EXAMINERS' FOLLOW-UP QUESTIONS

1   King George V went to Bognor to convalesce after his pneumonia, hence the addition of Regis to Bognor. Where would you send this patient to live permanently, if he could afford it?
2   Would steroids help him?
3   Why did he have a flapping tremor, and why were his aspartate transaminase and alkaline phosphatase elevated?
4   Do you think his emphysema is due to deficiency of $\alpha 1$ antitrypsin?
5   What would you do if his PCO_2 rose after admission to hospital?

D.G.J.

Confusion in an alcoholic

WHAT IS THE DIFFERENTIAL DIAGNOSIS?

1   Wernicke's encephalopathy
    Acute alcohol toxicity
    Cerebral trauma
    Alcohol withdrawal
    Hypoglycaemia

The combination of acute confusion, ataxia, ophthalmoplegia, nystagmus and peripheral neuropathy suggests a diagnosis of Wernicke's encephalopathy. The patient had been drinking heavily for many years and had lived on an inadequate diet consisting mainly of carbohydrate. Acute toxicity needs to be considered — but there was no history of a recent heavy binge and the patient's breath smelt only slightly of alcohol. It is also important to consider trauma to the head and it must be remembered that alcoholics are particularly susceptible to subdural haemorrhage. In this patient's case there was no history of recent head injury nor were there any external signs of trauma. Neurological examination did not reveal evidence of raised intracranial pressure.

Acute confusion may be a presenting feature of one of the syndromes of alcohol withdrawal. It can follow a withdrawal fit and it may be a feature of delirium tremens in which case the patient is usually restless, pyrexial and shows evidence of perceptual disturbance, particularly in the visual modality. An alcoholic binge can also cause hypoglycaemia which may present with acute confusion.

WHAT ADDITIONAL INVESTIGATIONS WOULD YOU REQUIRE?

1   CT brain scan
This will help determine whether there is evidence of intracranial haemorrhage or other cerebral lesion. In this patient it showed slight cortical atrophy but no localised lesion.

2   Blood alcohol
The blood alcohol level in this patient was 10.5 mmol/l, within the legal limit for driving a motor vehicle.

3   Blood glucose
Following admission to the Accident and Emergency Department the

blood glucose was 6.0 mmol/l thereby excluding hypoglycaemia as a cause of the patient's symptoms.

4 Serum pyruvate
This is raised in Wernicke's encephalopathy because of deficiency of thiamine which is required in carbohydrate metabolism. A random specimen was reported as 112 mmol/l (normal fasting range 41–67 mmol/l).

WHAT IS THE FINAL DIAGNOSIS?

Wernicke's encephalopathy.

HOW WOULD YOU MANAGE THIS PATIENT?
The patient was given an immediate intravenous dose of 50 mg thiamine and admitted to an acute medical ward. Intravenous therapy was started with dextrose-saline solution and he was given high doses of intravenous B vitamins over the next five days. During this time there was a marked improvement in his condition. He became less drowsy, his speech became clearer and the abnormal ocular signs disappeared. However he remained disorientated in time and place and his memory impairment persisted — he could not recall details of recent events nor could he learn new information. He was continued on oral vitamins, rich in thiamine, and three weeks after admission his memory had definitely improved. He could orientate himself correctly and he had learned the identity of the nursing and medical staff treating him. An occupational therapy assessment showed he was capable of looking after himself independently. He was seen by a psychiatrist specialising in the treatment of alcoholism and two weeks later he was allowed home after an outpatient appointment had been made for him in the local alcoholism unit.

COMMENT

Acute confusion is common in chronic alcoholics and it has a variety of causes, each of which require specific management. Wernicke's encephalopathy occurs in alcoholics who neglect themselves and exist on a poor diet. It is due to deficiency of thiamine and the acute clinical condition results from pathological changes occurring in the mamillary bodies, walls of the third ventricle, peri-aqueductal grey matter, dorso-medial nucleus of the thalamus and cerebellum. The pathological changes take the form of oedema, hyperaemia and petechial haemorrhages. Of those brought to hospital approximately 15 per cent make a good recovery as occurred in this patient. The remainder go on to develop Korsakoff's syndrome once the acute confusion has been resolved. This is characterised by profound memory impairment and confabulation. Once the features of Korsakoff's syndrome are established a significant degree of recovery occurs in only a small proportion, probably less than 20 per cent.

It is always worth recommending life-long treatment with a multi-vitamin preparation, containing thiamine, whenever an alcohol-related illness is diagnosed.

EXAMINERS' FOLLOW-UP QUESTIONS

1 What other neuro-psychiatric complications occur in chronic alcoholism?
2 How would you manage a patient who develops delirium tremens?
3 What is the mechanism for hypoglycaemia precipitated by alcohol?
4 What proportion of patients in acute medical wards in British hospitals are thought to have alcohol-related problems?
5 What are the currently recommended safe levels of drinking for men and women?

G.G.L.

A student with jaundice

WHAT IS THE DIFFERENTIAL DIAGNOSIS?

1   Acute virus hepatitis
       Type A
       Type B
       Non-A, non-B
    Infectious mononucleosis
    Chronic autoimmune hepatitis
    Alcoholic hepatitis

In a young person the combination of a flu-like illness with anorexia, followed by jaundice with dark urine and pale stools, strongly suggests virus hepatitis. The increased serum aspartate transaminase, with only a slightly-elevated alkaline phosphatase, supports the diagnosis. The virus hepatitis might be type A (faecal spread), type B (blood spread) or non-A, non-B (blood or faecal spread).

The absence of sore throat and lymphadenopathy makes infectious mononucleosis unlikely. Chronic hepatitis (autoimmune) is unlikely in view of the male sex, the acute onset and the absence of splenomegaly.

Alcoholic hepatitis is unlikely at this age; in older patients who take excessive alcohol, exposure to the inexpensive alcoholic drinks of Spain would make this a diagnosis to be considered seriously.

WHAT ADDITIONAL INVESTIGATIONS WOULD YOU CONSIDER?

1   Hepatitis virus serological markers
Hepatitis A IgM antibody was present and this confirms the diagnosis of acute hepatitis A. This antibody appears with the onset of jaundice and has usually (but not always) disappeared by eight to nine weeks. The IgG antibody appears at about that time and persists indefinitely. If the IgG antibody is present, it could indicate either past or present infection with hepatitis A.

Hepatitis B surface antigen appears about seven days before the patient becomes jaundiced. It indicates present or past hepatitis B infection. It was absent in this patient. If acute hepatitis B is strongly suspected, and hepatitis B surface antigen is negative, the patient may be in the period when the surface antigen has been cleared but antibody to surface antigen has not yet developed. In this circumstance hepatitis B IgM core antibody will be found. It was not considered necessary to perform this investigation, as the patient had the IgM hepatitis A antibody.

There are no specific markers for the non-A, non-B group of viruses. Diagnosis is by exclusion of other causes of virus hepatitis, particularly types A and B.

2 Serum immunoglobulin G (IgG)
The value was 13 g/l (normal 5–15 g/l). This excludes chronic auto-immune liver disease.

3 'Monospot' screen for infectious mononucleosis
This is hardly necessary in this patient, but might have been requested at the first consultation, to exclude Epstein Barr virus infection, as results for the virus hepatitis markers are often slow to come through from the laboratory (the results for the hepatitis A IgM antibody might not have been known for a week or so). The Monospot test was negative.

4 Liver biopsy
This is not necessary for the diagnosis of patients with acute virus hepatitis.

WHAT IS THE FINAL DIAGNOSIS?

Acute type A virus hepatitis.

HOW WOULD YOU MANAGE THIS PATIENT?

Before treating the patient, it is probably more important to consider the protection of his close contacts. Immune serum globulin is effective in preventing or modifying type A virus hepatitis. If administered before, or within two weeks of exposure, in a dose of 0.02 ml/kg intramuscularly, it will prevent illness in 80–90 per cent of those exposed. It should be given as soon as possible to this patient's father, mother, younger brother and sister and to his girl-friend.

Hepatitis A infection never becomes chronic, and if the patient survives the acute attack, which is very likely, he will make a complete recovery. If his home surroundings are good, he may be treated at home. Whilst he feels ill, he should stay in bed, with bathroom privileges. When his condition improves, he may be allowed to be up and around the house, resting as much as possible. Convalescence is about twice the period of bed rest.

The traditional low-fat, high-carbohydrate diet is popular because it has proved most palatable to the anorexic patient. When the appetite returns, he may eat anything he fancies. Supplementary vitamins, aminoacids and lipotrophic agents are not necessary. Corticosteroids should not be given.

Following clinical recovery the patient should not be questioned too closely about symptoms and feelings of weakness, for a post-hepatitis syndrome can readily be induced by the physician. Exercise must be undertaken within the limits of fatigue. Alcohol is denied for six months: the patient often has little inclination for it and excessive consumption leads to relapse. An increase of serum aspartate transaminase for up to six months after the acute attack is not unusual, and does not imply chronicity.

COMMENT

Hepatitis A was the most likely diagnosis. This is usually contracted by faecal contamination of water, or by food being handled by someone incubating the disease. The camping holiday in Spain would provide a suitable background; shellfish might have been the vehicle.

Hepatitis B was much less likely. The patient was not a homosexual, he denied intravenous drugs, he had not received a blood transfusion nor had he had recent dental treatment.

Non-A, non-B hepatitis was possible and this accounts for about 15 per cent of cases of sporadic viral hepatitis in the United Kingdom. The attack was rather acute for this type, which is usually milder and with less deep jaundice. Non-A, non-B hepatitis is usually blood-borne, but can be water-borne, particularly in Pakistan and India. Chronic hepatitis commonly develops after non-A, non-B hepatitis.

EXAMINERS' FOLLOW-UP QUESTIONS

1 Why was urobilinogen absent from the urine at presentation?
2 Why did the patient lose weight?
3 Why was the white blood count $3 \times 10^9/l$?
4 How do clams spread hepatitis?
5 What other infections might this young man have acquired on a camping holiday in Spain?

S.S.

Increasing malaise

WHAT IS THE DIFFERENTIAL DIAGNOSIS?

1   End-stage cirrhosis of the liver

The combination of mild jaundice, vascular spiders, palmar erythema, early hepatic encephalopathy (tremor, insomnia, poor memory) with ascites, hepatosplenomegaly, hypoalbuminaemia and a rise of serum transaminases could be explained by no other diagnosis.

WHAT ADDITIONAL INVESTIGATIONS WOULD YOU CONSIDER?

1   Prothrombin time and platelet count
The prothrombin time was 22 seconds with a control of 13 seconds. After vitamin K1 10 mg intramuscularly for two days, the value was 20 seconds. This value precluded liver biopsy which, in any case, would have been contraindicated by the gross ascites. The platelet count was $60 \times 10^9/l$. The thrombocytopenia and leukopenia were due to the enlarged spleen (secondary hypersplenism).

2   24-hour urine volume with electrolytes
The volume was 600 ml, containing 5 mmol sodium and 40 mmol potassium. This implies marked sodium retention with secondary hyperaldosteronism. The patient is unlikely to respond easily to therapy for the ascites.

3   Creatinine clearance
The creatinine clearance was 30 ml/min, a reduced value (normal 90–120 ml/min), which raises the possibility that the patient might develop the hepato-renal syndrome.

4   Urine culture
This was done to exclude a urinary tract infection as a cause of the decompensated hepatocellular function.

5   Sample ascitic fluid
About 50 ml were aspirated. The protein content was 10 g/l suggesting a transudate. The white cell count was 50/dl, all lymphocytes: this excludes 'spontaneous' bacterial peritonitis. Anaerobic and aerobic cultures were set up and tubercle bacilli sought by direct smear and by culture. Samples for routine bacteriology culture are best sent to the laboratory in blood culture bottles.

6 EEG

This showed a reduction in the mean frequency to 5 cycles/second (normal 8–13 cycles/second). Some slow waves were seen. These findings confirm early hepatic encephalopathy.

7 Upper gastrointestinal endoscopy

This showed large blue oesophageal and fundal varices, demonstrating that the patient has portal hypertension. The colour implies bleeding is not imminent.

8 Hepatic scan

There was poor uptake of the technetium isotope by the liver, but the large spleen showed marked uptake. This picture confirms chronic liver disease with splenomegaly. A localised filling defect was not seen.

9 Hepatitis B markers

Tests for hepatitis B surface antigen and hepatitis B core antibody were negative. A relationship of the cirrhosis to hepatitis B is highly unlikely.

10 Serum autoantibodies

Antinuclear, smooth muscle and mitochondrial antibodies were absent. This makes cirrhosis following an autoimmune chronic active hepatitis unlikely.

11 Serum alpha fetoprotein

The level was 4 IU/ml by radioimmunoassay (normal < 10 IU/ml). This is well below the level found in primary liver cancer.

12 Serum iron and ferritin

This man showed the picture of cirrhosis in whom the aetiology could not be determined by serological markers. He also had some testicular atrophy and the liver biopsy was not possible. Idiopathic haemochromatosis has to be excluded: he had a low serum iron and a normal serum ferritin.

WHAT IS THE FINAL DIAGNOSIS?

Cryptogenic cirrhosis of liver, with portal hypertension and hepatic failure. 'Cryptogenic' means 'of unknown aetiology'.

HOW WOULD YOU MANAGE THIS PATIENT?

The patient should be admitted to hospital. Routine oral ascorbic acid and vitamin B supplements are given. He should be maintained on an intake/output chart and the four-hourly temperature recorded. He should be weighed at the same time every morning. Serum electrolytes should be measured three times a week. Fluid intake should be restricted to one litre daily. The diet must be very low in sodium (less than 22 mmol daily). In view of the encephalopathy, dietary protein should be restricted to 40 g daily, increasing to 60 g as the clinical condition improves. A magnesium sulphate enema should be given on admission and oral lactulose ordered in a dose sufficient to ensure two semi-solid bowel motions daily. A diuretic may be required if bed rest, water and salt restriction fail to control the ascites. Amiloride is the diuretic of choice for a male cirrhotic, as it does not cause gynaecomastia.

COMMENT

The patient has liver failure and portal hypertension. Liver failure is shown by the skin changes, jaundice, encephalopathy, ascites and coagulation defects. Intrahepatic portal hypertension is shown by the dilated periumbilical veins, splenomegaly and oesophageal varices.

This patient's hepatic cirrhosis is of unknown aetiology. The cause might have been a past acute non-A, non-B virus infection but he had never received a blood transfusion. There are no laboratory tests for the non-A and non-B virus. The aetiology might be alcoholism, the patient having forsaken alcohol and 'forgetting' to give a history of it. The aetiology might be hepatitis B, the markers having disappeared from the circulation. The prognosis must be very guarded and treatment can only be directed towards 'patching up' a totally disorganised liver. Hepatic transplantation must be considered and this will depend upon such factors as psycho-social status. However, poor nutrition, age and reduced creatinine clearance made this patient a bad candidate.

EXAMINERS' FOLLOW-UP QUESTIONS

1   What are the factors precipitating decompensation in a patient with previously well-compensated hepatic cirrhosis?
2   Why does this patient have a low serum albumin concentration?
3   If the patient's fluid retention is not controlled by diet and diuretics, what measures would you consider?
4   Is this patient likely to develop renal failure? If so, discuss the mechanisms and treatment.
5   What factors determine the prognosis for this patient?

S.S.

Eye problems

WHAT IS THE DIFFERENTIAL DIAGNOSIS?

1　Graves' disease
　　Post-thyroidectomy hypothyroidism
　　Exophthalmos
　　Pretibial myxoedema
2　Diabetes mellitus
3　Macrocytosis
　　Hypothyroidism
　　Pernicious anaemia

The patient has had a thyroidectomy and has now developed the symptoms of hypothyroidism, as well as the signs of thyroid eye disease, and pretibial myxoedema. She has a macrocytosis (MCV 102 fl) which could be due to either hypothyroidism or pernicious anaemia. The random urine test revealed glycosuria: does she have diabetes mellitus?

WHAT ADDITIONAL INVESTIGATIONS WOULD YOU CONSIDER?

1　Serum thyroxine, free thyroxine index, and thyrotropin (TSH) concentration

The serum thyroxine concentration was 42 nmol/l which is low (normal range 58–128 nmol/l) and the free thyroxine index was also low at 37 (normal range 52–142). The serum TSH concentration was elevated ($>$ 100 mU/l, normal $<$ 5 mU/l), confirming the diagnosis of primary hypothyroidism.

2　Thyroid autoantibodies

Both antithyroglobulin and the antimicrosomal antibodies were present in high titre (1:10^5 and 1:10^6, respectively). These results confirm that the primary hypothyroidism is due an autoallergic process.

3　Serum B12 concentration

The serum vitamin B12 concentration was normal at 210 ng/l (normal 160–925 ng/l). This result excludes pernicious anaemia as the cause of the macrocytosis. A mild macrocytosis is common in myxoedema, but the serum folate should also be checked (it was normal). The patient has normal liver function tests, but the γ-glutamyl transpeptidase should be checked as a screen for alcoholism. The patient was not haemolysing: the reticulocyte count was 0.8 per cent (normal less than 2 per cent).

4 Fasting blood glucose

The fasting blood glucose concentration was 9.3 mmol/l, which confirms the diagnosis of diabetes mellitus. Diabetes mellitus is now defined by the measurement of a fasting blood glucose of greater than 8 mmol/l, or a blood glucose of greater than 11 mmol/l two hours after a 75 g oral glucose load.

5 Thyroid stimulating antibody

Although measurement of this antibody is helpful in the overall assessment in the underlying pathological process of the disease distant to the thyroid gland, it does not play a critical role in making a decision about management. Thyroid stimulating antibody is present in sera from patients which Graves' disease and is believed to be the cause of hyperthyroidism. Sera from patients with pretibial myxoedema, but not exophthalmos alone, almost invariably have a thyroid stimulating antibody. This antibody's activity is expressed as the ability of a serum to displace radio-labelled thyrotropin bound to receptors on the thyroid follicular cell membranes. This patient's serum inhibited 80 per cent of thyrotropin binding to thyroid membranes. The assay of this antibody is carried out in only a few specialist centres.

WHAT IS THE FINAL DIAGNOSIS?

Graves' disease with post-thyroidectomy hypothyroidism, and delayed onset of exophthalmos and pretibial myxoedema. The patient also has diabetes mellitus.

HOW WOULD YOU MANAGE THIS PATIENT?

The hypothyroidism should be treated with oral thyroxine replacement, usually for life. The therapeutic dose varies between 100 and 200 μg daily, taken as a single dose in the morning. The dose is regulated by assessing the patient's clinical response to thyroxine, and the suppression of the elevated serum TSH concentrations.

Mild exophthalmos due to Graves' disease does not require treatment. However, if it is severe and progressive the patient should receive a large dose of oral steroids (initially 80–120 mg of prednisolone/day). This patient has exposure keratitis and is unable to close her eyes — she may require a high dose of steroids.

Pretibial myxoedema only requires treatment if it is severe. It may respond to local injections of a steroid, such as triamcinolone, but systemic steroids usually do not help.

The patient has mild diabetes mellitus but she is not ketotic. She should be treated by dietary carbohydrate restriction; oral hypo-glycaemic agents should only be used if the diet fails. If the patient is given systemic steroids a deterioration of diabetic control should be anticipated.

COMMENT

Graves' disease consists of three major components: thyroid dysfunc-tion, eye disease and skin disease.

Although hyperthyroidism is the usual manifestation of the thyroid abnormality, patients may be euthyroid or hypothyroid. Histological examination of the thyroid glands invariably reveals evidence of auto-allergic inflammation.

The natural history of each of the three components of Graves' disease is independent from the other two. Although all three may have a simultaneous onset, exophthalmos or pretibial myxoedema may be separated from thyroid dysfunction by several years. Similarly, the treatment of hyperthyroidism in Graves' disease does not alter the onset or severity of either the eye or skin disease.

EXAMINERS' FOLLOW-UP QUESTIONS

1   Could this patient have become hypothyroid, even if she had not received surgery and had only been treated with drugs?
2   What drugs are used in the treatment of thyrotoxicosis?
3   Why is diabetes often associated with Graves' disease?
4   What are the advantages and disadvantages of radioactive iodine, when compared with partial thyroidectomy, for thyrotoxicosis?
5   Is there any hazard associated with the start of thyroxine replace-ment therapy for myxoedema, especially in older patients?

P.D.

A sick sailor

WHAT IS THE DIFFERENTIAL DIAGNOSIS?

1 Mumps meningo-encephalitis
  Tuberculous meningitis
  Pyogenic meningitis
  Uveo-parotitis
    Sarcoidosis

The patient has fever and meningism. Obviously an infectious meningitis must be excluded as soon as possible, but papilloedema is unusual in meningitis unless there is a space-occupying lesion. This patient also has bilateral parotitis and uveitis. The inflamed eye makes mumps unlikely but, particularly in a West Indian, it raises the possibility of sarcoidosis with an aseptic meningitis. Sarcoidosis could be a cause of the raised ESR and serum calcium.

WHAT FURTHER INVESTIGATIONS WOULD YOU CONSIDER?

1 CT brain scan
The patient has papilloedema in the left eye and the right disc cannot be examined. An urgent brain scan is required before a lumbar puncture is performed. The brain was completely normal.

2 Lumbar puncture
There was a clear tap of fluid under slightly raised pressure (19 cm fluid, normal < 15 cm). There were 12×10^6 lymphocytes/l (normal $0–5 \times 10^6$/l), the protein was elevated at 0.7 g/l (normal 0.15–0.4 g/l), but the blood and spinal fluid glucose concentrations were similar (3.3 and 3.1 mmol/l, respectively). Gram and Ziehl Neelsen stains did not reveal pyogenic bacteria or mycobacteria.

These changes suggest a viral or aseptic meningitis.

3 Chest X-ray
There was bilateral hilar lymph node enlargement, with a smooth lobulated outline. There was no sign of a pulmonary infiltrate, nor evidence of focal or miliary tuberculosis.

4 Mantoux Test
Tuberculin (0.1 ml 1:10 000, intradermal injection) did not produce any reaction by 48 hours. However, the patient had already started treatment before the results of this test became available.

5 Kveim–Siltzbach skin test

Some 80 per cent of patients with hilar lymphadenopathy due to sarcoidosis have a positive Kveim–Siltzbach skin test when the injection site is biopsied four to six weeks after the intradermal injection. This would be of little help for the diagnosis of an acutely ill patient.

6 Serum angiotensin converting enzyme

The serum concentration of this enzyme provides a measure of the activity of sarcoidosis. The results of a blood test taken on the day of admission became available some 12 days later: 87 nmol/ml/min (normal 16–52 nmol/ml/min).

WHAT IS THE FINAL DIAGNOSIS?

Sarcoidosis, with associated aseptic meningitis, uveo-parotitis, irido-cyclitis, and hilar lymphadenopathy.

HOW WOULD YOU MANAGE THIS PATIENT?

The patient is acutely ill and requires urgent treatment with steroids. The final diagnosis has been achieved by a combination of physical signs (which can be explained by sarcoidosis), an abnormal chest X-ray and the exclusion of an infectious meningitis.

All the patient's symptoms and signs will respond rapidly to steroids — prednisolone 60 mg per day by mouth, or intravenously if the patient has difficulty with swallowing. In addition, the patient needs atropine eyedrops to rest the inflamed iris.

The dose of steroids should be reduced as soon as the patient begins to respond. All the abnormalities in the laboratory screening tests should resolve during treatment with steroids.

COMMENT

Saroidosis may involve any level of the nervous system: meninges or peripheral nerves may be infiltrated and facial paralysis is common. The more abrupt the onset of sarcoidosis, the better the response to steroids. This patient should recover completely. However, he should be followed-up: if his symptoms return, or if he develops progressive impairment of lung function, he may require further treatment with steroids.

EXAMINERS' FOLLOW-UP QUESTIONS

1   What causes of papilloedema might the CT scan have identified?
2   What are the common bacteria that cause pyogenic meningitis?

3 What antibiotics would you use for these bacterial infections?
4 How do you treat tuberculous meningitis?
5 What abnormalities of respiratory function may be found in patients with advanced pulmonary sarcoidosis?

D.G.J.

A bearded lady

WHAT IS THE DIFFERENTIAL DIAGNOSIS?

1 Polycystic ovary syndrome
  Androgen-secreting tumour (ovarian or adrenal)

The combination of amenorrhoea and hirsutes suggests androgenisation. This patient has mild androgenisation, as there is absence of acne, excessive libido or clitoral enlargement. Mild androgen excess suggests the diagnosis of polycystic ovaries, rather than an androgen-secreting tumour.

Congenital adrenal hyperplasia usually presents as sexual ambiguity at birth, but may rarely present in later life as virilism associated with primary amenorrhoea. This patient has menstruated, hence congenital adrenal hyperplasia can be excluded.

The contraceptive pill and hyperprolactinaemia are the other common causes of amenorrhoea, but neither is associated with androgenisation. The last common cause of hirsutism is Cushing's syndrome, but this patient does not have the typical fat distribution or soft skin.

WHAT ADDITIONAL INVESTIGATIONS WOULD YOU CONSIDER?

1 Plasma testosterone
The plasma testosterone is the major investigation for any woman with hirsutism. This patient's plasma testosterone was mildly elevated at 4.1 nmol/l (0.8–1.6 nmol/l). Patients with androgen-secreting tumours usually have much higher concentrations of plasma testosterone.

2 Abdominal ultrasound
Pelvic ultrasound is able to define accurately the size and shape of both ovaries. This patient's ultrasound examination revealed bilateral enlargement of the ovaries, the left being larger than the right. Androgen-secreting tumours of the ovary, like most primary tumours elsewhere, are not multiple.

Had the ovaries both appeared normal, the adrenals could have been assessed by ultrasound during the same examination, to exclude an adrenal mass.

3 Gonadotrophin releasing hormone
Patients with the polycystic ovary syndrome often have an exaggerated release of luteinising hormone following an intravenous injec-

tion of the releasing hormone (100 ug iv). This patient's serum luteinising hormone concentration rose to a maximum of 55 mu/l (normal less than 20 mu/l).

4 Laparoscopy

This investigation not only confirmed that the ovaries are both enlarged, but also allowed biopsy of an ovary. Histological examination of the biopsy revealed a thickened cortex and several immature follicles. These changes are characteristic of the polycystic ovary syndrome.

WHAT IS THE FINAL DIAGNOSIS?

Polycystic ovary syndrome.

HOW WOULD YOU MANAGE THIS PATIENT?

The aim of treatment is to control and reverse the hirsutes and to restore regular menstrual periods. This is achieved by the administration of the anti-androgen cyproterone acetate, from day 5 to day 15 of the menstrual cycle. The menstrual cycle is restored by the administration of a low-dose oestrogen 'contraceptive pill' or ethinyl oestradiol 50 ug, given from day 5 to day 25.

Since patients with polycystic ovaries often have anovulatory cycles, and since the contraceptive pill suppresses ovulation in any case, these patients have to come off the pill and cyproterone should they want to become pregnant. Furthermore, in view of their anovulation, they may require clomiphene or even gonadotrophin injections to induce the release of ova from the ovaries. It is difficult to achieve pregnancy.

COMMENT

The investigation and management of hirsutes provide a common but difficult clinical problem. The rare causes of organic hirsutism (ovarian or adrenal tumours, or congenital adrenal hyperplasia) must be eliminated. The tumours are resected surgically, but congenital adrenal hyperplasia responds dramatically to cortisol suppression.

EXAMINERS' FOLLOW-UP QUESTIONS

1 Does surgery have any place in the management of these patients?
2 What are the mechanisms underlying the pathogenesis of congenital adrenal hyperplasia?

3   How does clomiphene exert its biological effect?
4   Which ovarian tumours are likely to secrete androgens?
5   What are the hazards of oral contraception?

P.D.

A psychiatric problem

WHAT IS THE DIFFERENTIAL DIAGNOSIS?

1   Cushing's syndrome·
    Hypertension
    Mild diabetes mellitus
    Drug-induced hyperprolactinaemia and obesity
    Simple obesity with polycystic ovaries

The combination of rapid, progressive weight gain, widespread striae, myopathy, hirsutes and amenorrhoea suggests the diagnosis of adrenocortical hyperfunction, and androgenisation. This patient's combination of symptoms and signs is best explained by the presence of Cushing's syndrome. This clinical conclusion is supported by the presence of a hypokalaemic alkalosis and glycosuria on the screening tests.

WHAT ADDITIONAL INVESTIGATIONS WOULD YOU CONSIDER?

1   Plasma and urinary cortisol
Plasma cortisol estimations at 9 am and midnight may reveal loss of the normal circadian rhythm. However, the stress of hospital admission may make interpretation of this test difficult. This patient's cortisols were elevated: 210 and 306 nmol/l, (normal less than 170 nmol/l at 9 am, and less than 120 nmol/l at midnight).

The 24-hour urinary free cortisol excretion was also elevated: 1543 nmol (normal less than 290 nmol/24 h).

2   Dexamethasone suppression tests
Dexamethasone 0.5 mg six-hourly for 48 hours suppresses normal cortisol secretion, assessed by either a morning plasma cortisol or 24-hour urinary free cortisol.

This patient's cortisol secretion was not suppressed indicating hypersecretion of adrenal steroids, with the loss of normal feedback control. However, the cortisol secretion was suppressed by dexamethasone 2 mg six-hourly for 48 hours. The response to this four fold rise in dexamethasone dose suggests that the cortisol is not coming from an autonomous adrenal tumour.

3   Abdominal ultrasound
Ultrasound can determine whether there is bilateral adrenal hyperplasia, or whether there is a unilateral adrenal tumour. This patient had bilateral enlargement of the adrenals.

4 Abdominal CT scan

Computerised axial tomography can also be used to obtain a non-invasive view of the adrenals. However, this is not necessary if ultrasound provides a clear image of the adrenals.

5 Plasma adrenocorticotrophic hormone

Although the 9 am sample for ACTH may be within the normal range (10–80 ng/l), the midnight sample is invariably raised if there is an ACTH-secreting pituitary tumour (normal less than 80 ng/l). The ACTH concentrations may be extremely high if there is ectopic production by a tumour (oat cell carcinoma or carcinoid tumour).

6 Selective adrenal catheterisation

This is rarely required. It is indicated if there is no suppression of cortisol secretion by high-dose dexamethasone, and ultrasound or CT scanning have failed to identify an abnormal adrenal.

The venous blood from both adrenals can be analysed for plasma cortisol concentration, in an attempt to determine which adrenal is secreting the cortisol.

7. Skull X-rays

X-rays of the pituitary fossa are performed to determine the size of the pituitary gland. Enlargement of the sella turcica is found in only 20 per cent of ACTH-secreting pituitary tumours. This patient's X-ray was normal.

WHAT IS THE FINAL DIAGNOSIS?

Cushing's disease — bilateral adrenal hyperplasia, secondary to a pituitary ACTH-secreting tumour.

HOW WOULD YOU MANAGE THIS PATIENT?

There are two management aims for this patient: firstly, rapid control of the adrenal hypersecretion to restore normal metabolism; secondly, definitive treatment of the ACTH-secreting pituitary adenoma.

Metyrapone will control the adrenal hypersection. Metyrapone is an enzymatic inhibitor of cortisol synthesis which, when given at the appropriate dose of 750 mg six-hourly, will control or even obliterate cortisol secretion. Replacement oral cortisol therapy (using 30 mg of cortisone daily) is often given at the same time as metyrapone, to prevent an Addisonian crisis.

The pituitary tumour is best eliminated by either external irradiation, which destroys the neoplastic tissue over a period of several months, or by the transsphenoidal surgical removal of the adenoma. The choice of technique depends upon the experience available in a particular centre.

COMMENT

Simple obesity is often confused with Cushing's syndrome. Although any fat person may have striae, patients with simple obesity do not have the characteristic fat distribution of Cushing's syndrome, nor the thin skin. The combination of obesity and hirsutes makes Cushing's syndrome more likely, particularly if there is a proximal myopathy. The other differential diagnoses to be considered are depression and alcoholism. The finding of a macrocytosis or a raised γ glutamyl transpeptidase would favour the latter diagnosis.

EXAMINERS' FOLLOW-UP QUESTIONS

1 Can Cushing's syndrome present with schizophrenia?
2 Why did this patient have difficulty in climbing stairs?
3 What is the mechanism underlying excessive hair and amenor-rhoea in this patient?
4 Would bilateral adrenalectomy be an acceptable therapeutic measure for this patient?
5 How would you recognise an Addisonian crisis?

P.D.

189

A painful eye

WHAT IS THE DIFFERENTIAL DIAGNOSIS?

1   Subarachnoid haemorrhage
     Berry aneurysm of circle of Willis
  Glaucoma
  Meningitis
  Diabetes mellitus
  Cavernous aneurysm of carotid artery
  Sinusitis

The history and signs are strongly suggestive of subarachnoid haemorrhage from a berry aneurysm of the circle of Willis (posterior communicating aneurysm). The initial retro-orbital pain and vomiting would be caused by initial minor leakage from the aneurysm affecting the 3rd nerve in close relation to the posterior communicating artery.

Severe pain and involvement of the pupil distinguish this from other causes of 3rd nerve palsy in adult life (eg diabetes, giant cell arteritis, arteriosclerosis). Lumbar puncture at this stage may be normal, or may show mild xanthochromia, or blood-staining. Hospital admission is required urgently before rebleeding occurs.

After a latent interval, usually one to two weeks, rupture of the aneurysm occurs with severe (often fatal) subarachnoid haemorrhage. The mortality is 30 per cent in the first week. Note that the rupture is often related to exertion (straining or coitus) and the pain may be felt in the neck rather than the head. Vomiting is very common, and the level of consciousness becomes progressively impaired. Retinal haemorrhages, especially subhyaloid, are a feature of severe subarachnoid haemorrhage. The neck is usually rigid, the limbs are flaccid, reflexes often depressed and plantar responses extensor. The blood pressure may be raised and there may be glycosuria.

Glaucoma may cause pain and vomiting especially in elderly patients; the vision is blurred, the pupil is oval and non-reactive, but there is neither ophthalmoplegia nor retinal haemorrhage.

Meningitis is unlikely because of the absence of fever and neck stiffness when she developed a 3rd nerve palsy.

Diabetes may cause a sudden 3rd nerve palsy with some pain but the pupil is usually normal. It must be excluded by routine tests.

An aneurysm of the cavernous portion of the carotid usually occurs in elderly women and causes a 6th nerve palsy in addition to a 3rd nerve palsy and partial trigeminal sensory loss. The pupil is usually small. This aneurysm rarely ruptures to cause a subarachnoid haemorrhage.

Acute sphenoid sinusitis may cause pain and a 3rd nerve palsy, but the onset would not be so acute and meningeal signs would be absent.

WHAT ADDITIONAL INVESTIGATIONS WOULD YOU CONSIDER?

1   Lumbar puncture
This showed evenly blood-stained fluid under increased pressure, confirming the diagnosis of a subarachnoid haemorrhage.

2   CT brain scan
This showed blood in the basal cisterns but no intracerebral haematoma. Extensive bleeding in the basal cisterns is usually associated with arterial spasm.

3   Cerebral angiography
This is always necessary as a preliminary to surgery, but may be postponed until the patient is fit for operation. In this case, right carotid angiography after three days showed a small saccular aneurysm projecting backwards near the termination of the internal carotid. Oblique views were necessary to show the neck of aneurysm. No spasm was present.

4   Platelet count, prothrombin time, bleeding time
Any tendency to spontaneous haemorrhage must be detected before surgery: all this patient's clotting studies were normal.

WHAT IS THE FINAL DIAGNOSIS?

Berry aneurysm of right carotid artery (posterior communicating aneurysm), causing a subarachnoid haemorrhorage and 3rd nerve palsy.

HOW WOULD YOU MANAGE THIS PATIENT?

In a young previously fit patient, who recovers full consciousness after subarachnoid haemorrhage from a berry aneurysm in this situation, the best treatment is surgical obliteration of the aneurysm by the clipping of its neck. The timing of the operation is important and the surgeon should be consulted before angiography. In unoperated patients there is a grave risk of rebleeding usually after 10–14 days; operation is best performed within a few days of the patient becoming alert and orientated. If extensive spasm is shown on angiography, or CT scan shows haematoma or infarction, further delay may be advisable.

After clipping, a second angiogram is often performed to confirm obliteration of the aneurysm. The 3rd nerve palsy usually recovers in a few weeks but recovery may be incomplete and the pupil may remain paralysed.

COMMENT

In most patients with a subarachnoid haemorrhage four vessel angiography is necessary to detect the bleeding aneurysm. In 10–20 per cent of patients multiple aneurysms are found. In this patient the 3rd nerve palsy clearly indicated the site and side of the bleeding vessel, and vertebral angiography was omitted. If no aneurysm is found, patients are normally kept on strict bed rest for 4–6 weeks.

Paroxysmal hypertension resulting from a phaeochromocytoma or from vasopressor drugs may sometimes provoke subarachnoid haemorrhage.

EXAMINERS' FOLLOW-UP QUESTIONS

1   Why is it important to feel the femoral pulse?
2   Why was the blood pressure raised after the second (severe) haemorrhage?
3   Why does diabetic 3rd nerve palsy leave the pupil unaffected?
4   A tendency to lid retraction on downward gaze is a common sequel to 3rd nerve palsy due to an aneurysm (pseudo von Graeffe's sign). What is the cause of this?
5   How may aspirin alter haemostasis?

R.W.R.R.

Continuing dyspepsia

WHAT IS THE DIFFERENTIAL DIAGNOSIS?

1   Recurrent peptic ulceration
    Carcinoma of the stomach
    Chronic pancreatitis
    Cholelithiasis
    Depression

The patient has continuing dyspepsia, but cannot explain the exact nature of the ulcer operation. If the pain is associated with that operation, this raises three main possibilities: that the surgeon only controlled the haemorrhage and did not perform a definitive ulcer-healing operation; that he did perform such an operation, but it failed; that a gastric malignancy was found at that operation, which has now recurred.

Alternatively, the present symptoms may be unrelated to the surgery: chronic pancreatitis and cholelithiasis are common causes of severe epigastric pain, but the patient has an iron deficiency anaemia which is not associated with either of these conditions. Depression commonly presents as epigastric pain, especially when the patient complains of unremitting symptoms.

WHAT ADDITIONAL INVESTIGATIONS WOULD YOU CONSIDER?

1   Get the operation notes and histology
An unconventional 'investigation', but extremely important. The patient had a pyloric canal ulcer, which had penetrated into the pancreas. The antrum and ulcer were resected with difficulty, and a Polya reconstruction performed. Histology revealed chronic peptic ulceration, without evidence of malignancy.

2   Upper gastrointestinal endoscopy
Endoscopy is much better than radiology for the assessment of the operated stomach. The endoscopist reported 'a massive anastomotic ulcer, with signs of recent bleeding'. Biopsies and cytology from the ulcer edge did not reveal malignancy.

3   Fasting plasma gastrin
430 pg/ml (normal < 80 pg/ml). Any recurrent ulceration following surgery must raise the possibility of hypergastrinaemia. The high fasting plasma gastrin is only found in three situations: pernicious

anaemia, the Zollinger-Ellison syndrome, and when a cuff of antrum is retained at the top of a Polya loop.

4 Pentagastrin test

Gastroenterologists almost never use acid secretion tests for everyday clinical problems, except when there is failed gastric surgery. As this patient has a raised fasting gastrin, it is most important to prove that he is secreting acid, and-does not have achlorhydria due to pernicious anaemia.

This patient's results for a standard pentagastrin test were basal acid secretion 37 mmol/h, peak acid output 44 mmol/h.

These results strongly suggest the Zollinger-Ellison syndrome, as not only is there massive gastric secretion in the basal state, but this is virtually unchanged by maximal stimulation with pentagastrin.

5 Technetium gastric scan

The patient could possibly have the extremely rare retained cuff of gastric antrum at the top of the Polya loop. If a remnant of antral mucosa is left in this position, its gastrin secreting cells are only bathed in alkali from the pancreas, which stimulates massive release of gastrin.

Intravenous technetium is taken up by gastric mucosa, and the abdomen is scanned with a gamma camera. This may show the independent cuff of gastric antrum at the head of the duodenal loop. This patient's gastric scan was normal.

6 Secretin provocation test

In a healthy subject, an intravenous bolus of 75 clinical units of secretin causes a rapid drop of plasma gastrin concentration. In a patient with the Zollinger-Ellison syndrome there is a further rise of fasting gastrin. This patient's fasting plasma gastrin concentrations were 490, 510, 514 pg/ml which rose after intravenous secretin to 540, 570, 590, 610, 490 pg/ml.

WHAT IS THE FINAL DIAGNOSIS?

Anastomotic gastro-jejunal ulceration, due to a gastrin secreting tumour (Zollinger-Ellison syndrome).

HOW WOULD YOU MANAGE THIS PATIENT?

The immediate problem is to control gastric acid secretion. Fortunately, most of these patients respond to an H_2-antagonist, usually at a higher dose than normal. The patient had already failed to respond to conventional doses of cimetidine, so the patient should be changed to a more potent H_2-antagonist regimen: for example, ranitidine 300 mg or famotidine 40 mg four times a day.

In future, the H^+, K^+–ATPase blocker omeprazole will probably be the treatment of choice (40–80 mg daily).

In order to check that the anti-secretory drugs are sufficient, it is best to pass a nasogastric tube during the daytime whilst the patient eats a normal diet, and takes the drugs. The pH should always be more alkaline than 1.8. The drugs should be increased until the acidity is controlled.

Having controlled the gastric hypersecretion, the patient may then be investigated at leisure to see whether there is a resectable pancreatic tumour.

Before H_2-blockers, the only surgical treatment was a total gastrectomy (to remove the target organ for the gastrin) and a total pancreatectomy: a combined procedure with considerable mortality, and later morbidity.

A modern alternative strategy is to attempt to localise the tumour before surgery. Arteriography, an abdominal CT scan, or even pancreatic ultrasound may help. However, the most rewarding examination is sampling of the gastrin concentration in the splenic and portal veins, following their transhepatic cannulation.

If a tumour can be found, resection is probably advisable as 60 per cent are malignant. If a tumour cannot be found, some would suggest a blind distal pancreatectomy and a highly selective vagotomy. However, the risks of such surgery make long-term treatment with a potent anti-secretory drug regimen an acceptable alternative.

COMMENT

The Zollinger-Ellison syndrome may present in one of three ways: firstly, as aggressive peptic ulceration, often associated with a surgical catastrophe (anastomosis breakdown or recurrent ulceration with bleeding); secondly, failure to respond to H_2-blockade, particularly if there is endoscopic-proven continuing ulceration despite six to eight weeks full-dose treatment; thirdly, diarrhoea probably due to excessive duodenal acid, which inactivates pancreatic enzymes and precipitates bile salts.

EXAMINERS' FOLLOW-UP QUESTIONS

1 How do the side-effects of cimetidine and ranitidine differ?
2 Give five reasons why a patient with a Polya gastrectomy may be iron deficient.
3 What are the indications for surgery after a haematemesis?

4 What other syndromes are caused by polypeptide-secreting tumours?
5 If this patient had a normal fasting gastrin, would you still recommend further surgery?

R.E.P.

Weight loss and stiffness

WHAT IS THE DIFFERENTIAL DIAGNOSIS?

1   Polymyalgia rheumatica
    Temporal (giant cell) arteritis
    Malignancy
    Depression
    Rheumatoid arthritis

The combination of proximal limb girdle pain and marked stiffness, associated with systemic symptoms, is strongly suggestive of polymyalgia rheumatica. Typically this is an illness of fairly acute onset. The normocytic anaemia, elevated ESR, and raised alkaline phosphatase are all in keeping with this diagnosis.

However all these findings may also be compatible with malignant disease. Her symptoms, occurring near to the time of the death of her husband, could be explained by depression alone, but her screening tests are abnormal.

The distinction between polymyalgia rheumatica and early rheumatoid arthritis may be extremely difficult and it may depend on continued observation of the patient.

WHAT ADDITIONAL INVESTIGATIONS WOULD YOU CONSIDER?

1   Temporal artery biopsy
A 3 cm length of temporal artery was removed under local anaesthetic. Histology was normal. A positive temporal artery biopsy is diagnostic, but unfortunately a negative biopsy does not exclude temporal arteritis.

2   Rheumatoid factor
There was no agglutination of immunoglobulin-coated latex particles.

3   Muscle enzymes and electromyography
Creatinine kinase and aldolase levels were normal, as was the electromyogram. In polymyalgia rheumatica no definite abnormalities of muscles have been documented.

4   Screen for malignancy
Chest X-ray, intravenous pyelogram, barium series, hepatic and pancreatic ultrasound were all normal. These investigations were not really justified. A better course of action would be to treat the patient

for polymyalgia rheumatica, and only to investigate further in the absence of a response to therapy.

WHAT IS THE FINAL DIAGNOSIS?

Probable polymyalgia rheumatica.

HOW WOULD YOU MANAGE THE PATIENT?

She was given prednisolone 20 mg daily, and responded dramatically. One week after starting steroids her symptoms had disappeared and her ESR had fallen to 40 mm/1st hour. During the next two months steroids were gradually reduced to 10 mg daily; she remained well and her ESR averaged 20 mm/1st hour.

Her prednisolone dosage was subsequently reduced by 1 mg each month. However four months later she complained of severe headaches and blurring of vision in the right eye. Her ESR had increased to 84 mm/1st hour and biopsy of her remaining temporal artery now showed giant cell arteritis. Prednisolone was immediately increased to 60 mg daily and again her symptoms quickly resolved.

Prednisolone was tapered to 10 mg daily over the next three months, but by this time she had become hypertensive and her skin was extremely fragile. Two months later she remained well but her ESR had risen from 30 mm to 60 mm/1st hour. It was not felt justified to increase her prednisolone in the absence of symptoms. One year later her ESR was 50 mm/1st hour and she was taking 5 mg prednisolone daily. She died shortly afterwards of a myocardial infarct. A postmortem showed atherosclerosis of the coronary arteries, and no evidence of an arteritis.

COMMENT

This patient illustrates many of the problems in the management of polymyalgia rheumatica. Diagnosis is usually confirmed initially by a response to steroids accompanied by a fall in ESR. Although late progression to giant-cell arteritis may occur in up to 40 per cent of patients, no predictive factors have been identified. Old people are particularly susceptible to the side-effects of glucocorticoids and the dangers of the disease have to be balanced against the dangers of the therapy. In this context it is probably not justified to treat the ESR alone, but to warn the patient that, at the earliest symptoms suggesting giant cell arteritis, steroids should be increased.

EXAMINERS' FOLLOW-UP QUESTIONS

1 What are the complications of giant-cell arteritis?
2 How is polymyositis differentiated from polymyalgia?
3 Does a normal ESR exclude the diagnosis of polymyalgia rheumatica?
4 Would this patient respond to a non-steroidal anti-inflammatory drug?
5 Does the raised alkaline phosphatase come from liver or bone?

M.J.W
G.R.V.H.

Progressive weakness

WHAT IS THE DIFFERENTIAL DIAGNOSIS?

1   Acute post-infective polyneuritis (Guillain-Barré syndrome)
    Poliomyelitis
    Acute multiple sclerosis
    Toxic neuropathy
    Metabolic polyneuropathy
      Diabetes
      . Porphyria
    High spinal cord compression

Rapidly progressive paralysis beginning in the legs and spreading to involve arms and face strongly suggests a polyneuritis, but if the face were spared a high cervical cord compression or demyelination would be possible. Note the emphasis on motor rather than sensory features — it may be difficult to exclude polio in an unvaccinated subject.

Acute multiple sclerosis in the brain stem would be likely not only to cause ocular palsy, nystagmus and to have more prominent sensory features, but also the reflexes would probably be increased and the plantar responses extensor.

Toxic polyneuropathy (eg organophosphorus, arsenic or thallium) usually has a much slower course but it may occasionally be acute; skin or hair lesions may give diagnostic clues. Porphyria may cause an acute polyneuritis, but there is usually a history of abdominal pain and psychiatric features. Diabetic neuropathy is occasionally acute, but is excluded by routine tests.

Acute polyneuritis may follow diptheria or mycoplasma infections, or infections with the cytomegalovirus, Coxsackie or Epstein Barr viruses.

WHAT ADDITIONAL INVESTIGATIONS WOULD YOU CONSIDER?

1   Lumbar puncture
Cerebrospinal fluid protein: 1.6 g/l (normal 0.15–0.4 g/l), containing no cells. A raised protein with normal cell count is characteristic of the Guillain-Barré syndrome, but can also be found in diabetic neuropathy.

2   Vital capacity
Daily investigation is necessary to assess the progress of respiratory weakness. At presentation this patient's vital capacity was 1.6 l (expected 5.3 l).

3 Nerve conduction studies (performed one week later)

The median and lateral popliteal nerve conduction velocity in motor nerves was 10 m/sec (normal 50 m/sec), with delayed and diminished sensory action potential from the finger. Marked slowing of nerve conductions suggests a demyelinating type of neuropathy such as the Guillain-Barré syndrome.

Toxic neuropathy tends to affect axons and it produces relatively little change in conduction velocity. If the pathological changes are confined to the nerve roots (polyradiculopathy), conduction in distal segments of peripheral nerve may be normal in the early stages of the illness.

4 Urinary porphobilinogen

This screening test for acute intermittent porphyria was negative.

5 Toxicity testing

To exclude heavy metal poisoning, specimens of urine and blood were stored for later analysis.

6 Viral studies

Paired serum specimens were tested against common viral infections (mumps, Echo, Coxsackie): they were negative. The Paul Bunnell test for infectious mononucleosis was also negative. Serological screening for HIV infection should be performed in any patient in a high-risk category (do not forget counselling before the blood tests).

7 ECG

The ECG was normal, but occasional sudden deaths occur in patients with Guillain-Barré polyneuropathy, usually preceded by cardio-vascular signs of autonomic involvement. These may include any combination of tachycardia, bradycardia, hypertension or hypotension, and should be taken seriously. Temporary cardiac pacing is occasionally required.

WHAT IS THE FINAL DIAGNOSIS?

Acute post-infective polyneuritis (Guillain-Barré syndrome).

HOW WOULD YOU MANAGE THIS PATIENT?

The correct management of the ventilatory and bulbar weakness is of the first importance. Intubation and positive-pressure assisted respiration is usually necessary if the vital capacity falls below one litre. This patient's respiratory reserve is already severely compromised: his vital capacity is reduced from an expected volume of 5.3 to 1.6 l. Correct positioning of the patient, pharyngeal suction and a cuffed endotracheal tube to prevent inhalation of secretions are important. Weakness of swallowing may necessitate tube feeding. Facial weakness can cause exposure keratitis: eye care is important. Urinary catheterisation is usually necessary in severe cases.

The Guillain-Barré syndrome is self-limiting and the prognosis is good, provided complications are prevented. Corticosteroids are probably of no value, but plasmaphoresis may be tried in an early case where respiratory weakness is developing.

COMMENT

Most patients with Guillain-Barré syndrome begin to improve after one to two weeks, and thereafter recovery is rapid. Nerve axons are probably preserved and severe wasting usually does not occur. However, the occasional patient does develop distal muscle wasting, and recovery may then be incomplete. Obscure progressive or recurrent polyneuritis is usually found to be associated with malignant disease (carcinoma or lymphoma), or with a paraproteinaemia. Some of these may respond to treatment with steroids or to plasmaphoresis.

EXAMINERS' FOLLOW-UP QUESTIONS

1 What commonly-used drugs may cause polyneuritis?
2 What organism causes neuropathy by direct invasion of the nerves?
3 Why is the CSF protein raised in some types of polyneuritis?
4 What type of polyneuritis is characteristically preceded by paralysis of accommodation and by palatal weakness?
5 How may a British patient be exposed to polio infection?

R.W.R.R.

Palpitations and dizziness

WHAT IS THE DIFFERENTIAL DIAGNOSIS?

1 Panic attacks
   Paroxysmal supraventricular tachycardia
   Phaeochromocytoma

Panic attacks commonly present with dramatic physical symptoms which can mimic various medical conditions. Many of these symptoms can be reproduced by deliberate over-breathing. The patient may deny any associated anxiety or describe it as being secondary to the physical complaints. Panic attacks may be associated with symptoms of agoraphobia so the patient comes to lead a progressively more restricted life. It is important to remember that the physical examination may be completely normal in the case of paroxysmal cardiac arrythmias and also in patients with phaeochromocytoma.

WHAT ADDITIONAL INVESTIGATIONS WOULD YOU REQUIRE?

1 Precipitants and situation of attacks
When specifically questioned, the patient described her first attack as having occurred while waiting in a queue at a supermarket checkout. Other attacks had occurred in large department stores, in a cinema and on public transport. They had never occurred in her home. She had become very anxious at the prospect of going out alone to busy shopping areas and could only manage short walks to local shops. However she was able to venture further afield if her husband accompanied her.

2 Personal history
Just before the onset of her symptoms the patient had discovered that her husband was having an affair with another woman, but he claimed to have given up this relationship when his wife found out. The patient also reported that she had experienced school phobia during childhood and had attended a child guidance clinic for this reason.

3 Patient's alcohol history
She had been a very light drinker until the onset of her symptoms. However during the twelve months before her presentation she admitted that she had been drinking up to half a bottle of sherry daily. This relaxed her and made it easier for her to do her local shopping. This could explain her MCV of 101 fl.

4 ECG

This was normal, as was a 24 hour tape.

5 Urinary catecholamines

A 24-hour collection of hydroxymethylmandelic acid (5HMMA) was 22 μmol (normal range 16–48 μmol), excluding a phaeochromocytoma.

WHAT IS THE FINAL DIAGNOSIS?

Panic attacks with agoraphobia.

HOW WOULD YOU MANAGE THIS PATIENT?

Although the patient had some difficulty accepting a psychological explanation, she was relieved to learn that there was no cardiac disease or other serious physical abnormality. She was advised to stop drinking and was able to do this without difficulty in the anticipation that her symptoms would be helped. She was treated with imipramine, the dose being increased to 150 mg at night without any troublesome side effects. Her panic attacks became much reduced in frequency and intensity, but she remained agoraphobic and was unable to go to busy shopping areas or to use public transport on her own.

She was referred to a clinical psychologist who devised a programme of behaviour therapy based on relaxation and systematic desensitisation. Within two months, this treatment had been successful so that the patient was able to lead an unrestricted life. The psychologist also saw the patient and her husband together for six sessions of sexual counselling, because it was learned that they had been having serious sexual problems for two years before the husband had an affair.

COMMENT

Panic attacks can occur in isolation or in association with agoraphobia. They may be precipitated by specific situations such as crowded shops or enclosed areas, or they may occur randomly in which case they are more difficult to treat with behaviour therapy. Some psychiatrists believe panic attacks represent a form of affective disorder, and this is at the basis of the use of antidepressant drugs.

EXAMINERS' FOLLOW-UP QUESTIONS

1 What is the derivation of the term 'agoraphobia'?
2 What other psychotropic drugs may be used in treatment?
3 Name some other common phobias.

4 What are the other physical manifestations of anxiety?
5 What are the hazards of using benzodiazepines in the management of patients with chronic anxiety states?

G.G.L.

Holiday stomach upset

WHAT IS THE DIFFERENTIAL DIAGNOSIS?

1   Coeliac disease
    Continuing enteric infection
    Crohn's disease

The chronic iron deficiency and the incomplete response to oral iron suggests a problem that pre-existed the holiday. The patient is on iron, and now has a macrocytosis (MCV 104 fl), which may be due to B12 or folate deficiency, a reticulocytosis, thyroid disease, liver disease or alcoholism, or a myeloproliferative disorder.

The acute stomach upset was probably an enteric infection due to poor hygiene or faecal contamination of the holiday water supply, but it may have uncovered underlying bowel pathology.

The normal sigmoidoscopy makes inflammatory bowel disease unlikely, unless the patient has Crohn's disease with rectal sparing. However, active Crohn's disease is also unlikely as the patient has a normal ESR.

Probably the most common adult presentation of coeliac disease is recurrent iron or folate deficiency; diarrhoea or steatorrhoea are much less common, but in adults they often follow an infectious insult to the gut.

WHAT FURTHER INVESTIGATIONS WOULD YOU CONSIDER?

1   Stool samples for culture and parasites
The stool contained neither pathogens nor parasites. *Giardia lamblia* can be found in the stool, but microscopic examination of duodenal juice is a more reliable way of finding the parasite. Alternatively, a therapeutic trial of either metronidazole 400 mg three times a day, or a single dose of tinidazole 2 g, may be reasonable for persisting 'traveller's diarrhoea'.

2   Prothrombin time
14 seconds (control 13 seconds). If malabsorption is suspected, vitamin K deficiency must always be excluded before performing a jejunal biopsy. A prolonged prothrombin time due to malabsorption of vitamin K will be corrected overnight following an intramuscular injection of vitamin K1 10 mg. If the prolonged prothrombin time is due to liver disease the response is slower and less complete.

3   γ glutamyl transpeptidase
The patient has a raised alkaline phosphatase: is it from bone or the biliary tract? This patient's γ glutamyl transpeptidase was 22 IU/l

(normal 10–48 IU/l), suggesting no problem in the biliary tract. The alkaline phosphatase came from bone, strongly suggesting osteomalacia, which was confirmed by a trephine bone biopsy. A skeletal survey was normal, with no sign of Looser's zones or pseudofractures.

4 Jejunal biopsy and duodenal aspirate

When the small bowel is biopsied using a Crosby capsule, a sample of the duodenal juice should always be inspected for parasites by immediate microscopy. This patient's duodenal juice contained no *Giardia*. However, the jejunal biopsy showed subtotal villous atrophy, an appearance characteristic of coeliac disease.

5 Barium follow-through X-ray

Interpretation of a barium follow-through may be difficult, particularly when there is a diffuse mucosal lesion. The radiologist reported a coarse, rather than feathery, jejunal pattern will some flocculation of the barium. There was no evidence of either Crohn's disease or lymphoma.

6 Three-day faecal fat

Although this patient had mild steatorrhoea (27 mmol/day, normal range < 18 mmol/day) the combination of the jejunal biopsy and barium follow-through provides sufficient evidence for a confident diagnosis of coeliac disease. The faecal fat estimation was unnecessary and unpleasant for both patient and laboratory worker.

8 Blood film, serum folate and vitamin B12

The blood film showed a macrocytosis with a right shift of the neutrophils. Howell-Jolly bodies indicated hyposplenism, commonly seen in coeliac disease. The patient's macrocytosis was due to folic acid deficiency (serum folate 2.6 μg/l; normal range 3–20 μg/l). Folic acid and iron are absorbed in the proximal small bowel, the main area of damage in coeliac disease. Although vitamin B12 deficiency can be found in untreated coeliac disease, this patient's serum B12 was normal (200 ng/l; normal 160–925 ng/l).

WHAT IS THE FINAL DIAGNOSIS?

Coeliac disease (gluten enteropathy).

HOW WOULD YOU MANAGE THIS PATIENT?

A coeliac must eat a gluten-free diet for the rest of his or her life. The diet is a major inconvenience as the only gluten-free cereals are rice and maize. Eating at home is relatively easy, but institutional or social eating are considerable problems. In the early months the patient will need not only the support of a dietician, but also the Coeliac Society. The latter keeps an up-to-date register of gluten-free proprietary foods, which allows the coeliac patient to enjoy a more normal and varied diet.

As the jejunal mucosa recovers, the iron and folate deficiency should correct. Many gastroenterologists prefer not to treat these deficiencies, as they provide a functional assessment of intestinal recovery. Similarly, the alkaline phosphatase should fall as the patient absorbs calcium and vitamin D normally.

After six months on the diet, the jejunal biopsy should be repeated and a gluten challenge considered. As transient villous atrophy may follow an infectious insult to the small intestine, a clinical and histological relapse of the coeliac disease following gluten challenge provides definite evidence of the benefit of a strict diet. Not every gastroenterologist recommends gluten challenge in the adult, but it is almost mandatory in a child with villous atrophy (where enteritis or milk allergy provide an important differential diagnosis for coeliac disease).

COMMENT

Coeliac disease may present as a failure to thrive in the recently weaned child, as a cause of malabsorption with steatorrhoea or diarrhoea, or as unexplained iron or folate deficiency anaemia. Most patients respond to a gluten-free diet; compliance to the diet can be a problem but even the most conscientious patients do not always respond. If they are malnourished and ill, oral steroids may be the only successful treatment.

The sudden deterioration of a coeliac, with abdominal pain, weight-loss or diarrhoea, may herald the presence of an intestinal lymphoma. An accurate diagnosis may require a laparotomy, producing sometimes difficult-to-interpret histology. The prognosis for such a lymphoma is extremely poor.

EXAMINERS' FOLLOW-UP QUESTIONS

1 What skin condition is associated with villous atrophy?
2 How would you distinguish bacterial contamination of the small bowel lumen from coeliac disease?
3 What immunisation would you recommend for the prospective holidaymaker to the Mediterranean?
4 What are the advantages and disadvantages of parenteral iron therapy?
5 Where is there a high prevalence of coeliac disease in Europe?

R.E.P.

Oliguria after multiple injuries

WHAT IS THE DIFFERENTIAL DIAGNOSIS?

1 Acute renal failure
   Rhabdomyolysis (crush syndrome)
   Acute tubular necrosis
      prolonged hypotension
      gentamicin toxicity
      septicaemia
2 Lower urinary tract obstruction

A period of profound hypotension may produce acute tubular necrosis particularly, as in this patient, where resuscitation and restoration of blood volume and blood pressure are delayed or incomplete. The physical examination is strongly in favour of extensive muscle damage with marked swelling of the lower limbs. Aminoglycosides can contribute to acute renal failure, particularly if given in normal doses at regular intervals to a patient with impaired renal function. However, three 80 mg doses of gentamicin would not be enough to produce renal damage.

WHAT ADDITIONAL INVESTIGATIONS WOULD YOU PERFORM?

1 Creatine phosphokinase
The diagnosis of the crush syndrome can be confirmed by the finding of a grossly elevated creatine phosphokinase (10 000 IU/l, normal < 50 IU/l), the enzyme being released from crushed and necrotic muscle.

2 Uric acid
A large amount of purines are released from damaged muscles and it is not uncommon to find a markedly elevated plasma uric acid in rhabdomyolysis. This patient's uric acid was 1.12 mmol/l (normal 0.1–0.4 mmol/l).

3 Urine myoglobin
Myoglobin is filtered very rapidly by the glomerulus as its molecular weight is less than that of haemoglobin. Urine can be tested for the presence of myoglobin by spectroscopic and chemical methods. Urine microscopy usually shows numerous casts in the acute renal failure of rhabdomyolysis, and there are often some red cells. Finding 'brown sugar' casts of myoglobin may suggest the diagnosis. Myoglobin not only forms renal casts, which contribute to renal failure by obstructing the nephron, but it is also directly nephrotoxic.

4 Leg arteriogram

Although the history suggests that compression may be the cause of the left lower limb ischaemia, rupture of the femoral artery may occur in blunt trauma. If there is any doubt about the leg's viability, an arteriogram should be performed. It is not uncommon for raised pressure in muscle compartments to reduce, or even abolish pedal pulses.

5 Urinary catheterisation and urine analysis

A urethral catheter should be passed to exclude rupture of the urethra and to obtain a sample of urine for analysis. Simultaneous plasma values should be obtained so that the urine-to-plasma ratios of urea and osmolarity can be calculated. The results obtained in this patient were as follows:

Urinary sodium: 80 mmol/l   Plasma sodium: 143 mmol/l
Urinary urea: 85 mmol/l   Plasma urea: 24.3 mmol/l
Urine osmolarity: 385 mosmol/l   Plasma osmolarity:
    301 mosmol/l

These figures give a urine/plasma urea ratio of about three, with a urine/plasma osmolarity ratio of little more than one. These results indicate established renal failure as the quality of the urine is poor: that is, akin to unaltered glomerular filtrate. This patient is unable to conserve sodium or make a concentrated urine with respect to plasma, despite clinical evidence of hypovolaemia. In patients with pre-renal renal failure (poor perfusion of otherwise normal kidneys), the urinary urea is 10–20 times the plasma urea, the urinary sodium is usually less than 10 mmol/l, and the urine/plasma osmolarity ratio is greater than 1.5. These general rules only apply to patients who are oliguric and not taking diuretics at the time the urine sample is taken.

The implication of this patient's results are that he will not respond to rehydration followed by diuretics. He is in established acute renal failure, and almost certainly will need a period of dialysis until kidney function returns.

WHAT IS THE FINAL DIAGNOSIS?

Crush injury: acute rhabdomyolysis producing acute renal failure.

HOW WOULD YOU MANAGE THIS PATIENT?

His biochemistry is seriously deranged and he is liable to have a cardiac arrest from the dangerous combination of hyperkalaemia and hypocalcaemia. He should receive the following intravenous treatment urgently:

1   10 ml 10 per cent calcium gluconate (which may need to be repeated several times).

2   50 ml 50 per cent dextrose with 20 units of soluble insulin.
3   50 ml of 8.4 per cent sodium bicarbonate.

His fluid depletion has not yet been fully corrected. The low haemoglobin and low plasma proteins suggest extensive sequestration of
sero-sanguinous fluid within the damaged muscle compartment. His
circulating blood volume should be expanded with a unit of whole
blood and sufficient plasma to restore his blood pressure and
peripheral perfusion.

After correction of his circulating blood volume a frusemide challenge may be given. If he does not respond to 80 mg frusemide given
intravenously, then 120 mg may be given as a further bolus. If no
response is obtained 1 g may be infused over four hours: deafness may
result if it is given faster. He is however unlikely to respond to a
diuretic challenge as his urine biochemistry suggests established
acute renal failure. A small proportion of patients may respond and
urine volumes may be restored although the quality of the urine often
remains poor for some days (so-called polyuric acute tubular
necrosis). Restoration of urine output is worthwhile as it makes
management easier: it allows fluid intake and facilitates feeding.

Given the severity of his injuries, and the potentially dangerous
biochemistry, dialysis should be started without delay. In the absence
of abdominal trauma peritoneal dialysis may be sufficient. However,
the uraemic state in a young muscular man with extensive soft tissue
injury and infection may not be controlled by peritoneal dialysis alone.
It would therefore be reasonable to insert a wrist arteriovenous shunt
as soon as possible, and start haemodialysis initially on a daily basis.
Recently the techniques of continous arteriovenous haemofiltration
(CAVH) and continuous arteriovenous haemodialysis (CAVHD) have
been introduced for the management of acute renal failure, particularly in the setting of the intensive care unit.

Further supportive measures must not be forgotten. Antibiotics
should be continued, with further doses of gentamicin being dictated
by blood levels. He should be given a diet containing at least 2000
calories/day to counteract the catabolic state that follows infection
and tissue trauma. Fluids and sodium and potassium intake should be
restricted.

It is likely that he will remain oliguric for two to three weeks. Urine
volume may well return before quality, and dialysis may need to be
continued after the start of a diuresis to maintain control of the
biochemistry.

COMMENT

Damaged muscle liberates creatine, phosphate, potassium, purines
and various organic acids. This accounts for the disproportionately
high levels of creatinine and phosphate, and the marked acidosis. The
slightly raised bilirubin and elevated liver enzymes reflect the

metabolism of released myoglobin together with the release of other tissue enzymes. Calcium is avidly bound to damaged muscle hence the initial very low plasma calcium. This man did well and his renal function returned in three weeks. However, at about the time renal function returned he became nauseated and developed red painful sore eyes. His plasma calcium had risen to 4.02 mmol/l. Late hypercalcaemia complicates the recovery phase of the crush syndrome. It is due to several factors including mobilisation of bound calcium from recovering muscle, restoration of 1:25 dihydroxycholecalciferol synthesis by the kidney, fall in plasma phophate as renal function recovers, and a slow resolution of secondary hyperparathyroidism which develops during renal failure.

EXAMINERS' FOLLOW-UP QUESTIONS

1   Why is myoglobin more damaging to the kidney than haemoglobin?
2   In what other clinical situations may myoglobin be released into the blood stream in sufficient amounts to produce acute renal failure?
3   Had this man been transferred to a casualty department immediately after his accident could anything have been done to prevent him from developing acute renal failure?
4   Can the polyuric phase, that follows acute renal failure, be dangerous?
5   What types of clotting problem might this patient develop in the days after admission to hospital?

P.S.

Depression and pleurisy

WHAT IS THE DIFFERENTIAL DIAGNOSIS?

1 Systemic lupus erythematosus
Systemic vasculitis
Bacterial endocarditis or brucellosis
Cytomegalovirus or Epstein-Barr virus infection
Lymphoma
Recurrent pulmonary emboli

This nursing sister's symptoms involve many organ systems and strongly suggest a connective tissue disease. Especially relevant is the past history of an autoallergic condition, idiopathic thrombocytopenic purpura. In a young woman systemic lupus is the most likely diagnosis; the history of a premenstrual exacerbation of symptoms is very characteristic.

Clinical distinction between systemic lupus and other connective tissue diseases, especially the systemic necrotising vasculitides, may be difficult and special investigations are required.

It is always important to consider chronic low-grade sepsis in the diagnosis of an illness involving many systems. The results of disseminated infection, emboli and the host's immune responses may mimic a primary connective tissue disease. However, the particular organ involvement in this patient would be unlikely to result from sepsis.

Malignancy, especially lymphoma, may prove an equally difficult differential diagnosis and should be suspected in the face of negative tests for the diseases discussed above.

WHAT ADDITIONAL INVESTIGATIONS WOULD YOU CONSIDER?

1 Differential white count and platelet count
The absolute lymphocyte count was $0.9 \times 10^9/l$ (normal $> 1.5 \times 10^9/l$) and platelet count $200 \times 10^9/l$. No atypical mononuclear cells were seen, reducing the likelihood of infectious mononucleosis due to either the Epstein-Barr virus or cytomegalovirus. Lymphopenia is a characteristic feature of systemic lupus erythematosus. A high white count in a patient with systemic lupus is unusual and suggests infection.

2 Urine microscopy and culture
No cells or casts were seen on microscopy of a freshly spun specimen

of urine; no organisms were grown. Nephritis is an important feature of many multi-system disorders and may be overlooked easily.

3 Blood cultures
Three sets of blood cultures grew no microorganisms.

4 Chest X-ray and ECG
Both were normal. Persistent bilateral pleuritic chest pain is most probably a primary feature of systemic lupus in this patient; however multiple pulmonary emboli can complicate this disease. If either the CXR or ECG had suggested pulmonary hypertension, or if the patient had become breathless, then pulmonary function testing, a ventilation-perfusion radionuclide lung scan, and possibly pulmonary angiography would have been indicated.

5 Antinuclear antibodies and DNA binding
Antinuclear antibodies were demonstrated by indirect immunofluorescence at a titre of 1:160. This test, although sensitive, has low specificity for systemic lupus. If positive it is worth proceeding to tests for antibodies to double-stranded DNA. A Farr radioimmunoassay for antibodies to DNA was positive at 90 per cent (normal DNA binding < 30 per cent; note that the normal range varies with assay system employed). This test has high specificity for systemic lupus erythematosus and confirmed the clinical diagnosis in this patient.

6 Complement profile
C4 levels and CH50 (a measure of the capacity of the patient's whole serum to haemolyse antibody-coated erythrocytes) were both moderately depressed. There is a loose correlation between disease activity and depression of complement levels. Patients with low complement levels should be monitored closely, but the levels do not necessarily signify renal disease.

7 Anticardiolipin antibodies
These antibodies, directed against phospholipids, are found in lupus (as well as in other diseases) patients where thrombosis is a major feature. High titres are associated with a tendency to recurrent thrombosis, recurrent abortions in those patients becoming pregnant, and thrombocytopenia.

Other features sometimes associated with anticardiolipin antibodies are migraines and livedo reticularis — both present in this patient.

8 C-reactive protein
This was measured by radioimmunoassay to be 2 μg/ml (not elevated). This acute-phase protein is not usually elevated in uncomplicated systemic lupus, however active the disease. In the presence of coexistent infection, C-reactive protein concentrations may rise dramatically; it can be a very useful test.

WHAT IS THE FINAL DIAGNOSIS?

Systemic lupus erythematosus, with pleurisy due to serosal involvement. Depression and migraine suggest probable central nervous system involvement; and lymphopenia and previous idiopathic thrombocytopenic purpura demonstrate haematological involvement.

HOW WOULD YOU MANAGE THIS PATIENT?

The problem in the management of patients with systemic lupus is to achieve the correct balance of treatment. Non-steroidal inflammatory drugs are useful in the control of musculo-skeletal symptoms. If marked systemic features are present, as in this patient, oral corticosteroid therapy is usually required. It is seldom necessary to use more than prednisolone 30 mg daily, unless a patient has severe disease. Steroids should be given as a single morning dose. As soon as clinical improvement is obtained, the dose can be tapered and often an alternate day regimen can be introduced. The patient should be prescribed the lowest dose of steroids consistent with symptomatic well-being and functioning of vital organs, particularly renal function in the presence of nephritis. DNA binding and the complement profile should be monitored, but they should not act as a direct guide to steroid therapy.

Antimalarial agents, such as hydroxychloroquine, may be useful for cutaneous and rheumatic manifestations of disease and may act as steroid-sparing agents. The potential ophthalmic complications of these drugs must be monitored, though they are extremely rare at the low doses that are now used.

Immunosuppressive agents, such as azathioprine, have a place in the management of patients with severe vital organ involvement. They are used as steroid-sparing agents in patients who require large doses of steroids to control disease activity.

Other forms of therapy, such as a high-dose 'pulse' methyl prednisolone or plasma exchange for fulminating disease, must still be regarded as experimental.

Beta-blockers, such as propranolol, are occasionally useful in the migraine of SLE, and, fortunately, infrequently pose a major problem in those SLE patients with mild Raynaud's.

In patients with high-anticardiolipin antibodies who have manifested thrombotic complications, long-term anticoagulation should be seriously considered.

COMMENT

This woman, in common with most patients with systemic lupus, responded rapidly to oral steroid therapy. Prednisolone was tapered over the two months after diagnosis to 10 mg daily: it was then found that her symptoms recurred when prednisolone was further reduced. On a daily dose of 10 mg alternating with 7.5 mg the patient remained well and she worked full-time. DNA binding and complement levels returned to normal over a period of several months.

EXAMINERS' FOLLOW-UP QUESTIONS

1 Should this patient be prescribed a contraceptive pill?
2 Define the terms 'specificity' and 'sensitivity' when applied to a diagnostic test.
3 What are the adverse effects of immunosuppressive drugs and how should they be monitored?
4 Is hydralazine contraindicated in the management of hypertension in patients with systemic lupus?
5 What type of liver disease is associated with a high-titre of anti-nuclear antibodies?

M.J.W.
G.R.V.H.

Backache

WHAT IS THE DIFFERENTIAL DIAGNOSIS?

1 Ankylosing spondylitis
  Reiter's disease or reactive arthritis
  Psoriatic arthropathy
  Intervertebral disc prolapse

The nocturnal component, with early morning stiffness, in this patient's back pain strongly suggests an inflammatory condition. A co-existent history of iritis and heel pain makes the diagnosis of ankylosing spondylitis almost certain.

There is broad clinical overlap between several conditions associated with ankylosing spondylitis, and spondylitis may precede other manifestations of these diseases. Examples are psoriasis and inflammatory bowel disease. There was no history of antecedent enteric or urethral infection to suggest a reactive arthritis.

WHAT ADDITIONAL INVESTIGATIONS WOULD YOU CONSIDER?

1 Sacro-iliac joint X-ray
The sacro-iliac joint margins were indistinct and there was periarticular bony sclerosis, confirm the diagnosis of sacro-iliac arthritis.

2 Lumbar spine X-rays
Lateral X-rays showed squaring of the anterior vertebeal corners and there was calcification of the anterior longitudinal ligament. The apophyseal joints were not fused. These features are suggestive of ankylosing spondylitis.

3 Heel X-rays
An early erosion was seen on the left calcaneum at the attachment of the plantar aponeurosis.

4 Chest X-ray
This was normal.

5 ^{99m}Technetium bone scan
Increased isotope uptake was seen over the sacroiliac joints and at the left heel. In the presence of definite radiological abnormalities this test was not necessary. Sacroiliac joint scanning may be of value in patients with equivocal abnormalities on X-ray examination. It is a

test with low disease specificity. A positive scan implies osteoblastic activity, which is associated with many conditions.

6   HLA-B27 antigen

This histocompatibility antigen was shown to be present on the patient's lymphocytes by a microcytotoxicity test. In this patient the test was superfluous as the pre-test probability of disease was greater than 90 per cent, and either a positive or negative test result for the presence of HLA-B27 antigen would not significantly influence the post-test probability. HLA-B27 antigen identification is of most use in patients in whom the pre-test disease probability is about 50 per cent.

WHAT IS THE FINAL DIAGNOSIS?

Ankylosing spondylitis with extra-articular involvement: iritis and plantar fasciitis.

HOW WOULD YOU MANAGE THIS PATIENT?

Good symptomatic relief may be expected from a non-steroidal anti-inflammatory agent, such as indomethacin, prescribed in full dosage.

There is no known way of preventing disease progression, and the second line drugs used in rheumatoid arthritis (gold, penicillamine or hydroxychloroquine) have not been shown to be effective for the axial disease of ankylosing spondylitis. Recently, methotrexate has been claimed as effective in aggressive systemic seronegative 'spondyl-arthropathy', that is, where peripheral joints are actively involved.

Maintaining a posture of spinal extension, rather than flexion, is of the greatest importance. This can be encouraged by a regular pro-gramme of spinal extension exercises, with instructions in physio-therapy classes. A firm mattress, with a single pillow to prevent excessive neck flexion, and chairs with good back-support all help to preserve a satisfactory posture.

Although systemic corticosteroids have no place in the manage-ment of ankylosing spondylitis (except in severe associated uveitis), intra-articular steroids may be helpful. Steroid injections into painful tendon insertions may be of particular value.

Spinal radiotherapy has been abandoned in view of the long-term risks of malignancy, but local radiotherapy may have a place in the management of intractable heel pain.

Arthroplasty may be necessary when the hips and knees are affected severely.

COMMENT

There is wide clinical overlap between the seronegative (lacking rheumatoid factor) arthritides. That genetic influences are important has been made clear by the strong linkage between the possession of HLA-B27 and the tendency to develop ankylosing spondylitis. Widespread clinical evidence of active inflammatory disease may not be reflected in abnormalities of blood tests. Although the ESR is usually elevated, a normal ESR may coexist with active ankylosing spondylitis.

EXAMINERS' FOLLOW-UP QUESTIONS

1 What are the chances of this man's children developing ankylosing spondylitis?
2 What are the cardiac complications of ankylosing spondylitis?
3 What is reactive arthritis, and with which micro-organisms has it been associated?
4 Will a colectomy control the ankylosing spondylitis that may be associated with ulcerative colitis?
5 Can a patient with active peptic ulceration have an anti-inflammatory drug?

M.J.W.
G.R.V.H.

A mite too small

WHAT IS THE DIFFERENTIAL DIAGNOSIS?

1   Asthma
    Cystic fibrosis
    Bronchiectasis
    Ascaris lumbricoides infestation
2   Atopic eczema

With a clinical history of breathlessness aggravated by exercise or infection, together with a nocturnal cough, asthma must be the most likely diagnosis. The presence of eczema makes this diagnosis even more probable.

Cystic fibrosis remains a possibility, although the patient has no symptoms (apart from his small size) to suggest pancreatic insufficiency.

Bronchiectasis could cause this patient's symptoms, but he had no history of a severe episode of pneumonia, nor of pneumonia complicating whooping cough or measles.

Ascaris lumbricoides migrates through the intestinal wall, passing to the pulmonary circulation and entering the airways; it is a rare cause of asthma.

WHAT ADDITIONAL INVESTIGATIONS WOULD YOU CONSIDER?

1   Blood film
The peripheral blood contained eight per cent eosinophils. In a 12-year-old boy this finding supports the diagnosis of either asthma or a parasitic infection.

2   Chest X-ray
The chest was hyperinflated. The rib cage silhouette was square and the sides of the thorax parallel. The diaphragms were depressed to the 11th rib, the muscle reflections of the right diaphragm visible, and the upper lobe blood vessels distended.

3   Peak expiratory flow rate
The patient's peak flow was only 100 l/min, but after inhaling salbutamol this improved to 160 l/min, demonstrating reversible airways obstruction.

Had the peak flow been normal, it would have been worth exercising the patient for six minutes, when a reduction of at least 15 per cent would suggest an asthmatic tendency.

4 Skin tests

Using a range of immediate skin prick test antigens, the doctor should note weals, pseudopodia and surrounding flares at 15–20 minutes, fading after 60–90 minutes. Providing the control test is negative, a 15 mm weal surrounded by erythema constitutes a positive test. However, the size of the weal does not correlate with the severity of symptoms that may be provoked by an individual antigen. This patient showed grass pollen allergy, but was negative to horse antigens.

5 Sputum cytology

The patient's sputum contained eosinophils, but no mycelial elements of *Aspergillus fumigatus* were seen.

6 Sweat test

The patient's sweat sodium concentration was normal. This excludes the diagnosis of cystic fibrosis.

7 Stools for parasites

There was no evidence of an *Ascaris lumbricoides* infestation.

WHAT IS THE FINAL DIAGNOSIS?

Asthma, with associated flexural eczema.

HOW WOULD YOU MANAGE THIS PATIENT?

He would undoubtedly respond well to systemic steroids, but this could retard his growth even further.

He has shown an immediate improvement after inhaling salbutamol, and initially it would be worth following his response to regular treatment. Probably the best regimen for a child is to use a Rotahaler, inhaling 200 μg of salbutamol powder four times a day. The patient could be provided with a peak flow meter to monitor his progress.

If the asthma persists, he could try prophylactic therapy with sodium cromoglycate 20 mg three to four times daily, again as an inhaled powder. If sodium cromoglycate is ineffective, the patient could try an inhaled steroid: beclomethasone or betamethasone. A more severely affected child may need salbutamol, and also either cromoglycate or steroids. Theophylline should be considered before oral steroids are started.

The flexural eczema should respond to a weak hydrocortisone cream, but it would be worth searching for the sensitising agent. Depending on the site, it may be provoked by clothing, detergents, or nickel sensitivity. Detective work may be required by the patient as well as the doctor.

COMMENT

This patient needs encouragement, and should not be prevented from leading a normal life. He can continue to play rugby, and should continue horse-riding, as long as it is certain that episodes of asthma are not precipitated by the horse itself. Children with stubborn childhood asthma have later become Welsh Rugby Internationals, Captain of England at cricket and have even won an Olympic Gold Medal for running!

EXAMINERS' FOLLOW-UP QUESTIONS

1 What do you know about the use of nebulised salbutamol?
2 This patient's skin tests show that he is allergic to grass pollens; should he receive a course of desensitisation injections?
3 How would you manage an acute attack of asthma?
4 What happens to the blood gases during the development of a severe attack of asthma?
5 What industrial allergens may provoke occupational asthma?

D.G.J.

Chinatown blues

WHAT IS THE DIFFERENTIAL DIAGNOSIS?

1   Pulmonary tuberculosis
    Carcinoma of bronchus
    Bronchiectasis
2   Diabetes mellitus

The patient is obviously ill with a respiratory illness. The screening tests show a considerable systemic response with a normocytic anaemia and a raised ESR. In a patient from Hong Kong, tuberculosis must be the most likely diagnosis. However, carcinoma of the bronchus could also produce this picture. Bronchiectasis only accounts for the purulent sputum, not the systemic illness. The patient has glycosuria without ketones: mild diabetes is likely.

WHAT ADDITIONAL INVESTIGATIONS WOULD YOU CONSIDER?

1   Chest X-ray
There was bilateral upper lobe fibrosis, with a possibility of cavitation in the right upper lobe.

2   Tomography of the lung apices
There were several small cavities in the right upper lobe — an abnormality that strongly suggests active pulmonary tuberculosis.

3   Sputum examination
The patient is producing copious purulent sputum. An emergency examination of the sputum for tubercle bacilli is justified, especially if it avoids the admission of 'open' pulmonary tuberculosis to a general medical ward.

The Ziehl-Neelsen stain revealed that the sputum contained acid-and-alcohol-fast bacilli. After culture for six weeks M. tuberculosis was isolated; antibiotic sensitivities were available after a further six weeks — the organism was sensitive to all standard drugs.

4   Tuberculin test
A tuberculin test (0.1 ml 1:10 000 intradermally) produced a brisk 17 mm diameter erythematous reaction at 48 h. This test is unnecessary if the sputum contains tubercle bacilli, unless one suspects an associated immune deficiency.

5 Glucose tolerance test

The patient's fasting glucose was 9.3 mmol/l, rising to 13.2 mmol/l 120 minutes after 75 g glucose. Both of these results are above the defined limits for the diagnosis of diabetes mellitus (8 and 11 mmol/l respectively.)

WHAT IS THE FINAL DIAGNOSIS?

Pulmonary tuberculosis, and non-ketotic diabetes mellitus.

HOW WOULD YOU MANAGE THIS PATIENT?

The patient should stop working in the restaurant and be admitted to hospital, particularly as he has inadequate home conditions.

The patient's illness must be reported to the community physician; the patient's fellow inmates at the lodging house, and colleagues at work, should be screened without delay for tuberculosis. Screening should include a tuberculin test and chest X-ray.

The patient should be treated with daily rifampicin, isoniazid and ethambutol. All three should be continued until the organism is known to be fully sensitive; pyrazinamide or ethambutol can usually be stopped at that stage, approximately three months after starting treatment. The patient should continue with rifampicin and isoniazid for nine months.

Satisfactory progress and antituberculous chemotherapy should be assessed by conversion of the sputum to negative, disappearance of symptoms, rising weight and haemoglobin, a falling ESR, and continuing improvement on the chest X-ray. The final chest X-ray should show only vague bilateral apical fibrosis.

The patient appears to have maturity-onset diabetes mellitus; despite the stress of his pulmonary tuberculosis he is not ketotic. He should be treated with a controlled carbohydrate intake and an oral hypoglycaemic· agent. His impotence was not due to diabetic autonomic neuropathy: when his tuberculosis was controlled his potency returned. He must stop smoking.

COMMENT

Tuberculosis may masquerade as many other diseases. The diagnosis may be missed if the specialist fails to recognise the masquerades in other systems. Thus, tuberculosis may present with such varying diagnoses as pericarditis, Crohn's disease, pyelonephritis, salpingitis, intracerebral space-occupying mass, osteomyelitis, or even breast cancer.

Tuberculosis should always be considered in any inflammatory or infectious condition, especially in migrants from Pakistan, India, East

Africa and the Far East. Even in the indigenous British population, one should be alert to a grandparent's 'bronchitis', which may disseminate tuberculosis to an infant with diastrous consequences.

EXAMINERS' FOLLOW-UP QUESTIONS

1 What do you know about *Mycobacterium avium intracellulare*?
2 What screening procedures would you adopt to monitor toxicity due to either ethambutol or rifampicin?
3 What is the interaction between rifampicin and the oral contraceptive pill?
4 What other respiratory disorders cause finger clubbing?
5 What are the indications for BCG vaccination?

D.G.J.

Prolonged ill health

WHAT IS THE DIFFERENTIAL DIAGNOSIS?

1   Chronic renal failure
      Proximal myopathy
      Peripheral neuropathy
2   Acute renal failure
3   Carcinoma (for example, colon) with obstructive renal failure
4   Pernicious anaemia
5   Hypothyroidism
6   Diabetes mellitus and renal failure

The clinical presentation of renal failure is often vague and non-specific. One important decision that has to be made when a patient with severe impairment of renal function is first encountered is whether the patient has acute or chronic renal failure. The long history of symptoms, the anaemia and biochemical evidence of metabolic bone disease all suggest chronic rather than acute renal failure. The low plasma albumin reflects a prolonged period of poor nutrition rather than urinary loss. The absence of heavy proteinuria on urine analysis excludes the nephrotic syndrome.

Glycosuria with a normal blood sugar is not uncommon when there is renal impairment. It does not mean that the patient has diabetes mellitus; the glycosuria is the result of a combination of tubular damage and overperfusion of the few remaining nephrons, so that the capacity to reabsorb the filtered glucose load is exceeded. This patient's blood glucose was 5.2 mmol/l.

It is quite likely that the cause of this patient's renal failure is chronic and uncontrolled hypertension. The absence of fundal haemorrhages, exudates, or papilloedema, excludes accelerated phase hypertension. A chronic underlying glomerulonephritis cannot be excluded at this late stage.

The symptoms and signs of muscle weakness are characteristic of proximal myopathy. This is not uncommon in patients with a marked degree of osteomalacia associated with renal failure. The high alkaline phosphatase and low plasma calcium would also be compatible with osteomalacia. The low plasma calcium of renal failure can be explained in part by phosphate retention raising the plasma phosphate, but this was not the case in this patient. Lack of 1:25 dihydroxy cholecalciferol (produced in the kidney) is responsible.

The marked debility and weight loss raises the possibility of carcinomatosis. The renal failure could possibly be due to obstruction from malignant lymph nodes. An abdominal ultrasound (see below) would help.

Some of the features of advanced chronic renal failure are similar to pernicious anaemia (peripheral neuropathy and anaemia), but the anaemia of renal failure is normocytic and normochromic.

WHAT ADDITIONAL INVESTIGATIONS WOULD YOU CONSIDER?

1 High dose intravenous pyelogram (IVP)
From the evidence provided we cannot diagnose the cause of this man's renal failure. A carefully conducted, non-dehydrating, high dose intravenous urogram or an ultrasound examination will provide three important pieces of information: the size of the kidneys is crucial, as small kidneys imply chronic disease; the shape helps, as chronic pyelonephritis produces deep cortical scars which show as an irregular contracted kidney, particularly affecting the upper poles; finally, these investigations will almost invariably demonstrate obstruction to the urinary tract, if present. It is essential not to miss a treatable cause of renal failure, so an IVP and/or an ultrasound should always be performed. In advanced diabetic renal disease an ultrasound of the kidneys should be done and not an IVP as the X-ray contrast is nephrotoxic.

This patient's IVP showed two small smooth kidneys with no evidence of obstruction. This is the commonest finding in end-stage chronic renal failure, and is compatible with either long-standing chronic glomerulonephritis and/or hypertension as the cause of the renal failure.

2 Skeletal X-ray survey
Although the clinical picture and the biochemical data suggest osteomalacia, it is necessary to confirm the suspicion. Looser's zones (pseudofractures), which are bands of uncalcified bone matrix, may be seen in the ribs, across the pubic rami and in the neck of the femur as well as along the edge of the scapula. They may be absent, however, even in the presence of severe osteomalacia that can be demonstrated only by bone biopsy.

Osteomalacia frequently coexists with hyperparathyroidism in patients with chronic renal failure. A bone biopsy will accurately define the nature of the renal osteodystrophy, but for clinical management a skeletal survey is usually sufficient. Hyperparathyroidism is best detected by looking for tiny subcortical erosions along the radial border of the middle phalanges of the hands. It may be confirmed by finding an elevated parathyroid hormone.

3 Isoenzymes of alkaline phosphatase
Alkaline phosphatase may be derived from bone, gut or liver. It is therefore necessary to measure the isoenzymes of alkaline phophatase. This patient's alkaline phosphatase came entirely from bone.

4 Nerve conduction studies

If the clinical examination suggests a uraemic peripheral neuropathy it is helpful to document the severity with an objective test such as nerve conduction. This provides a method of assessing response to treatment and ensures that insidious progression does not occur.

5 Renal biopsy

So far, all that can be said about this patient is that he has chronic renal failure, with small smooth kidneys. The exact cause cannot be defined at this late stage. Indeed, were a renal biopsy to be performed it would reveal an 'end-stage' kidney, which would not be diagnostic. A renal biopsy is contraindicated at this level of renal function as it is dangerous and difficult, and will provide no useful information.

WHAT IS THE FINAL DIAGNOSIS?

Chronic renal failure with osteomalacia and peripheral neuropathy; cause uncertain.

HOW WOULD YOU MANAGE THIS PATIENT?

As this patient has developed some of the severe complications of long-standing renal failure, he needs to start dialysis as soon as possible. There would be little to be gained at this late stage from restrictive diets and complicated drug regimens. The main indications for starting dialysis in chronic renal failure include pericarditis, neurological symptoms or signs, uncontrollable hypertension, uncontrollable hyperkalaemia, gross fluid overload or gastrointestinal symptoms that cannot be controlled by diet alone.

His metabolic bone disease needs attention. The plasma phosphate must be controlled (aim at 1.5–2 mmol/l) either by dialysis alone or by the use of an oral phosphate binder (aluminium hydroxide) taken with meals. Hypophosphataemic osteomalacia will develop if the phosphate is reduced to subnormal levels. When the plasma phosphate has been controlled, 1 alpha hydroxylated vitamin D derivatives can be given, making sure that hypercalcaemia (or a calcium × phosphate product above 5) does not occur. Excessive vitamin D therapy can lead to hypercalcaemia and metastatic calcification. Within one month of starting 0.5 µg daily of 1 alpha hydroxycholecalciferol, this patient's proximal myopathy had resolved.

COMMENT

Metabolic bone disease is an almost universal accompaniment of chronic renal failure. Once the creatinine clearance falls much below

30 ml/min renal osteodystrophy starts. Diagnosis is difficult in the early stages, and bone biopsy may be required. Later skeletal changes can be readily detected on X-ray. There are four main reasons why metabolic bone disease is so common:

1 Phosphate is retained as renal failure progresses. Elevation of the plasma phosphate depresses the plasma ionised calcium.
2 The kidney's capacity to 1 alpha hydroxylate vitamin D is progressively lost with falling renal mass. Lack of 1:25 dihydroxycholecalciferol (the final active metabolite of vitamin D) leads to impaired calcium absorption from the gut and defective mineralisation of bone.
3 The low plasma calcium (reduced calcium absorption and elevated plasma phosphate) stimulates the parathyroid glands. Hyperparathyroidism develops with consequent activation of the osteoclasts and erosion of the bones.
4 The acidosis of chronic renal failure is partly buffered by bone, and this also has a demineralising effect.

EXAMINERS' FOLLOW-UP QUESTIONS

1 What are the most common causes of end-stage chronic renal failure?
2 What are the relative advantages and disadvantages of peritoneal dialysis versus haemodialysis?
3 To what extent would you expect this patient's anaemia to improve after starting dialysis?
4 Would this patient be suitable for a renal transplant?
5 What drug regimens do you use to treat 'mild' hypertension?

P.S.

Septic feet

WHAT IS THE DIFFERENTIAL DIAGNOSIS?

1   Diabetes mellitus
Acute ketoacidosis
Infected foot
Peripheral neuropathy
Peripheral vascular disease
Retinopathy
Nephropathy

The patient has had poorly controlled diabetes for many years and obviously has developed diabetic ketoacidosis, provoked by sepsis in the right foot. The sepsis is probably due to the dangerous combination of peripheral vascular and neurological disease in a diabetic.

She also probably has two of the other complications of diabetes: retinopathy and nephropathy.

WHAT ADDITIONAL INVESTIGATIONS WOULD YOU CONSIDER?

1   Blood glucose
The patient's blood glucose was 35.8 mmol/l.

2   Arterial blood gases
PO_2: 13.1 kPa
PCO_2: 3.2 kPa
pH: 7.12
The patient has a normal PO_2, but a subnormal PCO_2 due to hyper-ventillation and a low pH. The patient has a metabolic acidosis, which is moderately severe.

3   Microbiology
A culture should be taken from the infected foot. In addition, blood and urine cultures should be taken in any diabetic who is as ill as this patient. The culture from the foot later grew *Staphylococcus pyogenes*, sensitive to flucloxacillin, but this result would only be available 48–72 hours after admission.

4   Chest X-ray and ECG
They were normal, but they should always be performed in an ill diabetic, who is liable to suffer from either ischaemic heart disease or pulmonary infection.

5 X-ray of infected foot

The X-ray may show stress fractures associated with the loss of pain sensation in the foot. Osteomyelitis is relatively common in infected diabetic feet. However no change would be expected on X-ray if the infection has only been present for approximately one week. This patient's X-ray was normal.

WHAT IS THE FINAL DIAGNOSIS?

Diabetic ketoacidosis due to a *Staph. pyogenes* infection of the foot. The patient also has other complications of diabetes mellitus: retinopathy, peripheral vascular and nervous disease, and nephropathy.

HOW WOULD YOU MANAGE THIS PATIENT?

The patient requires immediate rehydration with intravenously-administered 0.9 per cent sodium chloride containing potassium chloride supplements. She may require four to six litres of intravenous fluid in the first 24 hours after admission. Soluble insulin should also be given intravenously (a bolus of 10 units initially, followed by a continuous infusion of five to ten units/hour) through an indwelling cannula in a different vein. The insulin and saline infusions should be stopped when the blood glucose has dropped to 8 mmol/l. They should be replaced by a single infusion containing glucose and insulin. A 500 ml bag of 5 per cent dextrose given intravenously every four hours, containing eight units of soluble insulin, will usually maintain a normal blood glucose until the patient restarts oral feeding and subcutaneous insulin injections.

The patient's acidosis does not require specific correction with a sodium bicarbonate infusion, which should only be given if the arterial pH is less than 7.10.

The infected areas of her feat should be cleaned with an antiseptic solution and a suitable antibiotic should be administered, particularly if the patient becomes febrile following rehydration. Whilst awaiting the results of the cultures, flucloxacillin would be a suitable 'blind' antibiotic.

This patient's diabetes has been unstable for some years. Twice-daily injections of insulin could be used in an attempt to achieve as good control as is possible, particularly in view of the patient's florid retinal microangiopathic complications.

Amongst all her diabetic complications, only retinopathy can be given specific help. After assessment of the retinal vessels by flourescein angiography, laser treatment could be used to burn the leashes of new blood vessels in the retina. Laser treatment has been shown to arrest or retard further deterioration of the proliferative retinopathy.

COMMENT

An attempt to produce 'tight' control of this patient's diabetes with multiple insulin injections only resulted in repeated episodes of hypoglycaemia, often occurring without warning. She was changed to a continuous subcutaneous infusion of soluble insulin using a portable pump. Near-perfect control of glucose homeostasis was achieved, confirmed by out-patient measurements of glycosylated haemoglobin (HbA_1) with the results in the range 7.2–8.3 per cent (normal range 5.5–8.5 per cent).

EXAMINERS' FOLLOW-UP QUESTIONS

1 Why is it inadvisable to rehydrate a patient with acute diabetic ketoacidosis using oral fluids?
2 What are the dangers of neovascularisation of the retina?
3 What are the other common ocular complications of long-standing diabetes?
4 What do you know about the 'human' insulin, new devices for insulin administration, and what regimen would be recommended for a newly-diagnosed 16-year-old diabetic?
5 How would you assess this patient's renal function?

P.D.

Impaired speech and memory

WHAT IS THE DIFFERENTIAL DIAGNOSIS?

1 Cerebral tumour
  Glioma
  Metastasis
  Meningioma
  Cerebral abscess
  Presenile dementia (Alzheimer disease)
  Cerebral thrombosis
  Subdural haematoma
  Chronic meningitis
  Neurosyphilis

This history of progressive dysphasia and memory loss, right homonymous field restriction and mild pyramidal signs on the right side suggest a lesion affecting the left temporal lobe. A glioma is the commonest lesion presenting in this way, but an abscess is a definite possibility in view of the past chronic otitis. Other types of cerebral tumour, such as metastases or a meningioma also require consideration.

Presenile dementia (Alzheimer disease) may present with dysphasia, but there should be no change in reflexes or visual field loss. The slowly progressive history does not suggest a vascular lesion, but a chronic subdural haematoma may have progressive symptoms. However, with a chronic subdural a history of headache would be expected, and dysphasia or field restriction would be unusual.

WHAT ADDITIONAL INVESTIGATIONS WOULD YOU CONSIDER?

1 Chest and skull X-rays
A chest X-ray is an essential first investigation to exclude a bronchial neoplasm, the commonest cause of cerebral metastases: it was normal. The skull X-ray showed sclerosis of the mastoid region on the left side, and pineal shift one centimetre to the right.

2 CT brain scan
This showed a mixed high and low density intracerebral lesion in the left temporal region, which enhanced after injection of contrast. There was surrounding low attenuation suggesting oedema and some midline shift. These are the typical features of a glioma, but this examination cannot reliably exclude an abscess or meningioma.

233

3 Left carotid arteriogram

This showed upper displacement of the middle cerebral branches by a temporal mass. This was a space-occupying lesion with many small abnormal blood vessels.

4 EEG

This showed slow wave abnormality in the left anterior temporal region.

WHAT IS THE FINAL DIAGNOSIS?

Probable malignant glioma, left temporal lobe.

HOW WOULD YOU MANAGE THE PATIENT?

Management involves some difficult decisions and is best taken in consultation with a neurosurgeon and with the patient's relatives. If the diagnosis is in doubt a biopsy may be advisable although this carries a risk of increasing the deficit, especially in a patient with dysphasia; for some small tumours in inaccessible sites stereotaxic biopsy offers some advantages. Combination radio and chemotherapy probably prolong life in most patients with malignant glioma, but the therapists usually require histological confirmation of the diagnosis before beginning treatment.

Dexamethasone reduces oedema around the tumour and often improves the symptoms temporarily. The symptoms of raised intracranial pressure usually respond dramatically.

Malignant gliomas infiltrate into the brain and cannot be excised completely. A temporal lobectomy, with an attempt at subtotal removal, would probably result in some prolongation of life but at the cost of severe aphasia and hemiplegia.

In this patient initial treatment with dexamethasone was followed by a biopsy of the lesion which confirmed a glioblastoma multiforme. The anterior part of the temporal lobe was excised to provide an internal decompression and part of the tumour was removed. A radical course of cobalt radiotherapy combined with chemotherapy was given, and steroids were continued in a small dose. The speech defect improved for some months. However, during the following year he again deteriorated with increasing right hemiparesis, dysphasia and occasional grand mal seizures.

COMMENT

Cerebral gliomas often present as epilepsy of late onset or as an advancing focal deficit. A CT brain scan enables a diagnosis to be made much earlier than previously. Since only palliative treatment is available, when the diagnosis of an infiltrating glioma is very likely and the patient has few symptoms, it is often better to treat the seizures and follow-up the patient in the clinic.

Since there is wide variation in the natural history and growth of glial tumours, surgery and radiotherapy may be postponed until symptoms are more severe, or until features of raised intracranial pressure appear. Steroids are very effective treatment for raised intracranial pressure (for example dexamethasone 4 mg four times a day) but very large doses tend to produce unacceptable side-effects.

EXAMINERS' FOLLOW-UP QUESTIONS

1 Which parts of the brain are most commonly affected by an otitic abscess?
2 Why does a temporal lobe tumour produce a visual field defect as an early sign?
3 What drugs are most effective for temporal lobe epilepsy?
4 Is sexual function affected in temporal lobe epilepsy?
5 Why did this patient have a dysphasia?

R.W.R.R.

Failed medical check-up

WHAT IS THE DIFFERENTIAL DIAGNOSIS?

1   Chronic hepatitis
      Hepatitis virus A, B, or non-A, non-B
      Autoimmune disease
      Wilson's disease
      Drug-related

On further questioning the patient gave a past history of syphilis at the age of 25, non-specific urethritis three times during the last three years, and gonorrhoea when aged 32. He also admitted to being an active homosexual. He indulged in group ano-oral sex sessions with as many as six partners in one night. This patient has hepatocellular disease evidenced by hepatomegaly, raised aspartate transaminase and bilirubin. In a practising homosexual this is likely to be of viral aetiology. AIDS could be a coincidental illness.

Hepatitis A, although common in homosexuals, is unlikely to be the cause of his present illness, as this infection never becomes chronic. Non-A, non-B hepatitis is, surprisingly, rarely spread by homosexual activities, certainly in the UK. Hepatitis B does have a major connection with the 'gay' scene. Hepatitis B infection becomes chronic in 10 per cent of those exposed. Hepatitis B seems the likely cause of this patient's chronic hepatitis.

WHAT ADDITIONAL INVESTIGATIONS WOULD YOU CONSIDER?

1   Hepatitis B viral markers
Hepatitis B surface antigen (HBsAg) was positive by radio-immunoassay. Hepatitis e antigen (HBeAg) was strongly positive, and e antibody (HBeAb) was negative. HBeAg is strongly connected with continuing viral replication, infectivity and ongoing disease. This patient's blood is very infectious and he is a danger to his sexual contacts.

Serum hepatitis B DNA polymerase is technically difficult to measure in the laboratory, and is costly, but it also reflects ongoing disease and infectivity. In this patient's case it was strongly positive.

2   Prothrombin time and platelet count
These were performed to assess whether it would be safe to perform needle biopsy of the liver. Both were within the normal range.

3 Needle biopsy of liver

This was performed to determine the nature of the hepatitis — whether it is chronic persistent, which is benign, or chronic active which is more serious and which may culminate in cirrhosis. The possibility of a cirrhosis already being present would also be determined.

In fact, the liver biopsy showed a normal zonal architecture, but the portal zones were expanded by a mainly lymphocytic infiltrate. There was increased portal-zone fibrous tissue. The limiting plate of liver cells was eroded by mild piecemeal necrosis of the hepatocytes. Orcein stains showed hepatitis B surface antigen present in a few liver cells. The picture was of a mild chronic active hepatitis without cirrhosis, probably related to hepatitis B.

4 Serum alpha fetoprotein screening

This was done to exclude primary liver cancer, a common complication of chronic hepatitis B infection. The level was within normal limits but the test should be repeated at approximately six-monthly intervals.

5 Antibody to HIV

This blood test was taken with the patient's permission, and it was negative.

WHAT IS THE FINAL DIAGNOSIS?

Mild chronic active hepatitis, due to hepatitis B virus.

HOW WOULD YOU MANAGE THIS PATIENT?

The patient must be warned that his blood is infectious and that he is liable to transmit hepatitis B to close contacts, especially sexual. Any regular sexual partner should be tested for hepatitis B surface antigen and if negative offered vaccination.

Therapeutic decisions are very difficult. The patient is virtually symptom-free and the liver biopsy shows only a mild chronic active hepatitis. It might be wise to wait six months and then repeat the HBeAb and HBeAg tests. Spontaneous conversion of e antigen positive to e antibody positive might have developed, and continued conservative management is then justified.

If, however, he remains e antigen positive, anti-viral therapy should be considered, with lymphoblastoid or recombinant interferon. Corticosteroids are contraindicated as they increase viraemia (evidenced by a rise in serum hepatitis B DNA polymerase and HBsAg) and cause most patients to remain e antigen positive. Every six months the patient should receive a medical check which should include biochemical tests of liver function, hepatitis B viral markers and alpha fetoprotein.

COMMENT

This patient shows many of the features of chronic hepatitis B infection. The condition is more common in males, the progress is slow and insidious, and the patient often has no symptoms. There is often no history of an acute attack of hepatitis. The serum bilirubin, transaminase and gammaglobulin values are rarely very high.

Interferon will convert HBeAg to HBeAb in about 70 per cent of those treated. HBsAg will probably remain positive. Serum biochemical tests will improve and liver biopsy show less active histology.

EXAMINERS' FOLLOW-UP QUESTIONS

1　What medical diseases, other than viral hepatitis, are associated with homosexual activity?
2　What is the nature of current hepatitis B vaccines — are they useful in promiscuous homosexuals?
3　Name the types of person in whom you would strongly consider hepatitis B as the cause of chronic liver disease.
4　What would make you suspect that a patient with a positive test for hepatitis B surface antigen had developed a primary liver cancer?
5　What is meant by vertical transmission of hepatitis B infection?

S.S.

A little stroke

WHAT IS THE DIFFERENTIAL DIAGNOSIS?

1 Transient ischaemic attacks (right middle cerebral artery territory)
   Right internal carotid artery stenosis
   Sensory epilepsy
   Right hemisphere tumour
   Polycythaemia
   Migraine aura

The rapid onset of a focal cerebral deficit with brief duration and full recovery suggests an ischaemic attack or focal epilepsy. A small cerebral haemorrhage may cause a single mild stroke, but does not cause repeated attacks. There was neither alteration of consciousness nor involuntary movements to suggest epilepsy, but it is impossible to exclude it on these grounds alone. Involvement of the arm, face and tongue on the left side give a precise localisation in the right Sylvian area and a past history of intermittent visual loss in the right eye (amaurosis fugax) is an important clue to internal carotid artery disease. Systolic bruits over the neck are in keeping with carotid artery disease; bilateral bruits suggest either disease on both sides or a more proximal source for the murmur. Delay in the superficial temporal pulse suggests right external carotid artery stenosis or occlusion. In migrainous patients an aura can sometimes occur without headache, but with a negative past history a diagnosis of migraine is highly unlikely.

WHAT ADDITIONAL INVESTIGATIONS WOULD YOU CONSIDER?

1 CT brain scan
This was normal, but should always be performed if available since some cerebral tumours, especially meningiomas, may present with intermittent focal symptoms.

2 EEG
This showed a mild excess of theta activity of the right side over the temporal leads. This is a non-specific finding consistent with ischaemia or tumour, but gives no positive indication of epilepsy.

3 Chest X-ray
Showed left ventricular enlargement and widening of aortic shadow.

An abnormal left cardiac border following myocardial infarction might have suggested a cardiac aneurysm, and a possible source of embolism to the brain.

4 ECG
Pathological Q waves and T wave flattening in leads 1,2 and aVl, consistent with old myocardial infarction, but excluding an aneurysm.

5 Red cell mass and plasma volume
The patient's haemoglobulin was 17g/dl and the packed cell volume was 0.52. The red cell mass was normal, but the plasma volume was reduced by 15 per cent. This indicates relative polycythaemia, probably a result of smoking.

6 Doppler study of the carotids
There was an abnormal velocity profile in the right internal carotid, with no reversal of flow in the supraorbital artery on compression of the superficial temporal artery. This confirms the site of the bruit is the internal carotid artery and suggests significant obstruction to flow.

7 Ophthalmodynamometry
Left 100/60, right 75/40. This shows a reduction in pressure in the right ophthalmic artery consistent with significant internal carotid artery stenosis.

8 Intravenous digital subtraction angiography of neck arteries
Showed severe stenosis at the origin of the right internal carotid; the left internal carotid showed mild irregularity and stenosis.

WHAT IS THE FINAL DIAGNOSIS?

Transient ischaemic attacks: right internal carotid artery stenosis due to atheroma, with coincident relative polycythaemia.

HOW WOULD YOU MANAGE THIS PATIENT?

The best treatment for a patient of this age (ie less than 65 years) with localised unilateral internal carotid artery stenosis, who is in a satisfactory cardiac state, is carotid endarterectomy. However, this can only be recommended if experienced vascular surgery is available. The risk of stroke is approximately five per cent per year, and it is possibly higher in the first few weeks after a transient ischaemic attack.

COMMENT

Where no vascular surgery is available, or where the patient is unfit for surgery, aspirin in low dose (75 mg/day) is recommended as a long-term preventive treatment. For patients seen immediately after the transient ischaemic attack (TIA) or whose clinical state is fluctuating, anticoagulation with warfarin for three to six months may be used. Control of severe hypertension is necessary before either aspirin or warfarin are given.

The atraumatic Doppler ultrasound of the carotids is useful as a screening test, and there is good correlation with angiography. However, Doppler cannot distinguish with certainty between subtotal occlusion and total occlusion, and it cannot detect mild degrees of carotid ulceration.

In a patient who has a minor stroke and is left with a persistent neurological deficit, carotid endarterectomy is deferred for six to eight weeks.

Hyperviscosity of the blood, whether due to true or relative poly-cythaemia, is associated with an increased risk of stroke. Regular venesection to keep the packed cell volume below 0.45 should be considered. This may not be necessary if the patient will stop smoking, as the packed cell volume may improve spontaneously.

EXAMINERS' FOLLOW-UP QUESTIONS

1 What are the risks and complications of anticoagulants in cerebral-vascular disease?
2 What may be seen in the retina during amaurosis fugax?
3 What cardiac conditions may give rise to cerebral embolism?
4 What is a lacunar stroke and how does it differ from a TIA?
5 What are the causes of polycythaemia?

R.W.R.R.

Haematuria

WHAT IS THE DIFFERENTIAL DIAGNOSIS?

1   Carcinoma of the prostate
    Occult malignancy
    Septicaemia: urinary tract infection
      Acquired haemorrhagic disorder
        Disseminated intravascular coagulation
        Circulating inhibitor/anticoagulant
        Thrombocytopenia
2   Anaemia
    Blood loss
      Haematuria
      Haemoperitoneum
    Marrow infiltration

Whatever may have happened in the earlier episodes of haematuria, it is apparent that he must now have a generalised coagulation disorder and/or thrombocytopenia. He has multiple bruises and oozes from venepuncture sites. In addition he could have a malignant ascites, but it seems more likely that he had bled into his abdominal cavity because of the speed with which he become uncomfortable and distended.

Blood loss, both within the body and through the renal tract, has been considerable. One of the most likely diagnoses would be a carcinoma of the prostate, but this was not confirmed by earlier investigations. A further possibility is that the transfusion of large amounts of bank blood caused a 'wash-out' phenomenon, with depletion of clotting factors and platelets.

WHAT ADDITIONAL INVESTIGATIONS WOULD YOU CONSIDER?

1   Blood film and platelet count

There was a neutrophil leucocytosis with an occasional myelocyte and toxic granulation. There was an occasional fragmented red cell, and a very rare nucleated red cell was found after a prolonged search of the blood film. The platelet count was $203 \times 10^9/l$ (normal 140–400 $\times$ $10^9/l$), and there were some large platelets present in the blood film.

It is difficult to say that he had a leucoerythroblastic blood picture as the early cells were very hard to find. The presence of large platelets suggests that young forms are circulating.

2   Coagulation screen

Prothrombin time: 22 sec   (control: 13 sec)

Partial thromboplastin time: 67 sec   (control: 40 sec)
Thrombin time: 25 sec   (control: 15 sec).
These tests show that there is an abnormality at all stages of the coagulation system. The first step is to see whether the abnormality is due to multiple deficiencies, or is due to the presence of either an inhibitor or anti-coagulant. Equal parts of the patient's plasma and the control plasma were mixed and retested; there was considerable correction, and one concludes that there is a deficiency of several coagulation factors, and no inhibitor of coagulation is present.

3   Fibrinogen and fibrin degradation products

Fibrinogen: 0.5 g/l   (normal: 2.0–4 g/l)
Titre of fibrin degradation products: > 128 < 256   (normal: < 8)
Ethanol gel test: positive

He had a low plasma fibrinogen, and has raised fibrin degradation products, and a positive ethanol gel titre (indicating the presence of soluble fibrin monomer complexes). This is definite evidence of disseminated intravascular coagulation.

4   Acid phosphatase

Acid phosphatase: 1.2 IU/l (normal < 1.8 IU/l). A normal acid phosphatase is found in 50 per cent of patients with prostatic carcinoma.

5   Abdominal ultrasound

'Ascites is present, consistent with a haemoperitoneum in view of high level of echo. The pancreas is normal.'

The patient has been complaining of abdominal distension and the clinical impression of ascites, probably due to an intraperitoneal bleed, has been confirmed. A diagnostic (20 ml) paracentisis would provide more reliable evidence of a haemoperitoneum.

6   Urological opinion

'His prostate is hard but I think some of it is due to calcification in the seminal vesicles. If you would like his prostate to be re-biopsied, we will be pleased to arrange this when his clotting is normal.'

7   Bone marrow aspirate and trephine biopsy

An aspiration sample from the sternum contained a scanty amount of normal marrow. Megakaryocytes were plentiful. There was an occasional suspicious cell. The sample from the iliac crest contained numerous clumps of malignant cells; their origin could not be determined.

This aspirate and trephine biopsy provided the first evidence of a disseminated malignant process, which is the most likely explanation for his haematological condition.

8 Oncology consultant

'I think this patient must have a biopsy of the prostate, as clinically this seems to be the most likely primary site. If positive, my first choice would be a bilateral orchidectomy, or alternatively stilboestrol therapy.'

WHAT IS THE FINAL DIAGNOSIS?

Chronic disseminated intravascular coagulation, due to probable carcinoma of the prostate.

HOW WOULD YOU MANAGE THIS PATIENT?

There are two issues to be considered; firstly, the control of the disseminated intravascular coagulation and secondly, the identification of the site of his primary tumour and its treatment. Any further invasive investigations cannot be undertaken until his coagulation disorder is brought under control.

In the first instance, he should be given a transfusion of concentrated red cells for his anaemia, 12 bags of cryoprecipitate as a source of factor VIII and fibrinogen. The 12 bags of cryoprecipitate should be repeated each day. Continuous intravenous heparin therapy should be started. A loading dose of 50–100 units per kg body weight is given, followed by a continuous infusion of 5–15 units per kg per hour. The dose of heparin is adjusted according to the clinical and laboratory response, aiming to keep the partial thromboplastin time between one-and-a-half and two-and-a-half times the control value.

After four days of this regimen there was no need for replacement therapy; platelets and fibrinogen were both normal and fibrin degradation products had fallen to the normal range. Two days later, and continuing on heparin therapy, a prostatic biopsy was performed. Histology confirmed that the prostatic tissue was infiltrated by moderately differentiated adenocarcinoma, with perineural and lymphatic infiltration.

COMMENT

Disseminated intravascular coagulation will often resolve when the underlying disorder, for example septicaemia, is treated effectively. It is uncommon to have to take such active measures as in this patient, but the haematuria and coagulation disorder had to be controlled first, before the underlying cause could be fully investigated and treated.

The management of disseminated intravascular coagulation is based on the laboratory results. By the time that the patient was fully investigated, he had already received several units of bank blood, which would cause a dilution effect and so make the results more difficult to interpret. It is a good principle to collect samples for coagulation tests *before* transfusing the patient.

It has been said that replacement therapy adds 'fuel to the fire', but clearly there are occasions when replacement therapy must be given to achieve haemostasis, particularly when there is continuing haemorrhage, as at operation. In this case, heparin was also given to break the vicious cycle of coagulation factor consumption. Interestingly, the platelet count was never reduced, and this suggests that endogenous platelet production was adequate to maintain platelet levels; large platelets were present on the blood film indicating that these were young platelets. It is worth noting that although the prostatic biopsy was done under full heparin cover there was some bleeding from both the urethra and the rectum, but it was not excessive.

EXAMINERS' FOLLOW-UP QUESTIONS

1 Would a bone scan have been helpful?
2 What clotting constituents are present in fresh frozen plasma?
3 What are the disadvantages of stilboestrol therapy for carcinoma of the prostate?
4 What methods are available for controlling heparin therapy?
5 What other conditions are associated with disseminated intravascular coagulation?

E.J.P.-W.

Index of Long Cases

Index of Final Diagnoses